The clinical placement

An essential guide for nursing students

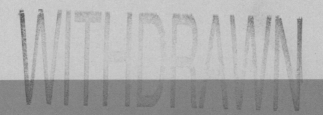

Dedications

This book is dedicated to my husband Garry,
and to my children Joel, Ben, Chelsea, Tyler and Madeline,
for reminding me what matters most in life;
and to my students, who continue to inspire me.
Tracy Levett-Jones

This book is dedicated to all students of nursing
(past, present and future):
a genuine treasure to human kind.
Sharon Bourgeois

The clinical placement

An essential guide for nursing students

Tracy Levett-Jones
Bachelor of Nursing Program Convenor and Senior Lecturer,
University of Newcastle

Sharon Bourgeois
Associate Head and Senior Lecturer,
School of Nursing, University of Western Sydney

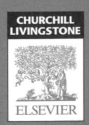

Sydney   Edinburgh   London   New York   Philadelphia   St Louis   Toronto

ELSEVIER

Churchill Livingstone
is an imprint of Elsevier

Elsevier Australia
(a division of Reed International Books Australia Pty Ltd)
30–52 Smidmore Street, Marrickville, NSW 2204
ACN 001 002 357

This edition © 2007 Elsevier Australia

National Library of Australia Cataloguing-in-Publication Data

---

Levett-Jones, Tracy
    The clinical placement: an essential guide for nursing students.

    1st ed.
    Includes index.

    ISBN-13: 978-0-7295-3798-8
    ISBN-10: 0-7295-3798-6.

    1. Nursing – Textbooks.   2. Nursing – Study and teaching.
    (Higher).   I. Bourgeois, Sharon.   II. Title.

    610.73

Publisher: Debbie Lee
Publishing Services Manager: Helena Klijn
Edited and project managed by Carol Natsis
Proofread and indexed by Forsyth Publishing Services
Design and typesetting by Modern Art Production Group
Printed in Australia by Ligare

Contents

About the authors

Tracy Levett-Jones

RN MEd&Work BN DipAppSC (Nsg)

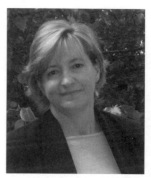

Tracy is Bachelor of Nursing Program Convenor and Senior Lecturer at the School of Nursing and Midwifery at the University of Newcastle. She holds the position of Honorary Research Fellow at the University of Southampton in the United Kingdom. Tracy has a broad clinical and educational background and has worked as a director of clinical education, nurse educator, new graduate program coordinator and women's health nurse. Her research interests include clinical education and competency development. Tracy believes that quality clinical placements are crucial to the development of competent and confident practitioners. Her doctoral studies explore the relationship between 'belonging' and the clinical experiences of nursing students in Australia and the United Kingdom.

Sharon Bourgeois

RN PhD MEd MA BA FCN FRCNA

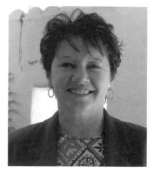

Sharon is Associate Head and Senior Lecturer at the School of Nursing at the University of Western Sydney. She has been involved in several leadership roles associated with clinical education for nursing students. She has also facilitated students' clinical and theoretical learning and supported registered nurses' educational development. Her formal research interests have focused on the discourses of caring, and identifying 'an archive of caring for nursing'. She has a strong interest in models of clinical education and the clinical learning environment. Sharon advocates that nurses embrace all elements of the professional role to enhance and promote care.

Introduction

There is plenty of evidence, anecdotal and empirical, to suggest that clinical placement experiences can be both tremendous and terrible. This book will help you to appreciate and capitalise on the tremendous, and dodge or ride out the terrible, in what is sure to be one of the most exciting journeys of your life.

The aim of this book is to guide you on your clinical journey. It provides our shared viewpoints, based on many years of experience with students in clinical and academic settings. However, there are many other viewpoints, perspectives and opinions that are equally valid, and we encourage you to talk to academic and clinical staff, educators, fellow students, friends and family about your placement experiences.

The ultimate goal of clinical education is the development of nurses who are confident and competent beginning practitioners. A positive and productive clinical placement experience is pivotal to your success. This book encourages you to use your clinical placement as an opportunity to develop the skills and knowledge that underpin quality practice, and to appreciate the clinical environment for the wonderful learning experience that it provides.

While deceptively simple, this book explores complex clinical learning issues. Although it is written primarily for nursing students, it will also be of interest to anyone involved in the clinical education of undergraduate students. Academics, clinical educators, facilitators, clinicians, mentors and managers will find the information it contains useful as a stimulus for dialogue and debate in tutorials and debriefing sessions. The book's interactive style and 'plain English' language approach are designed to engage with active readers and to encourage them to integrate the material into their practice.

How to use this book

Each chapter consists of a number of different sections. Within these sections theory is interwoven to explain core principles. **Stories and scenarios** appear throughout the book to help you relate theory to the reality of practice. **Something to think about** boxes provide words of wisdom to reflect on and valuable snippets of advice. **Coaching tips** allow you to apply what you learn to your clinical experiences.

The book is set out so that you can read from front to back. However, you may feel that some parts are more relevant to you than others, in which case you can simply skip back and forth.

Chapter 1 sets the scene by focusing on the 'rules of engagement' in complex clinical environments. The clinical context and culture are described and coaching tips provided to help you navigate your way successfully through this dynamic and exciting journey.

Chapter 2 provides insights into the 'great expectations' placed upon nursing students by patients, clinicians and the nursing profession as a whole. Armed with a clear understanding of what is required as you traverse the clinical learning milieu, your chances of success will be multiplied.

Chapter 3 gives a practical and positive description of how to behave and act within clinical environments. Tips for maximising learning opportunities are provided, along with strategies for dealing with difficult and challenging situations.

Chapter 4 focuses on the beliefs, attitudes and values that underpin successful clinical performance and encourages you to think about and reflect on your experiences in ways that are meaningful and relevant.

Chapter 5 looks at the ways nurses define and promote their profession through effective communication and gives advice on how to interact with clients and colleagues.

Chapter 6 is a compilation of sections written by expert nurses. We are delighted to include the viewpoints and perspectives of people from a wide cross-section of nursing specialties as they introduce you to the particular learning opportunities and challenges inherent in diverse clinical areas. Of course, we haven't been able to cover every clinical specialty, but we hope that the selection included opens your eyes to the wonderful opportunities available to nursing students and to graduates.

At the end of each chapter we have included **reflective thinking activities**. We encourage you to undertake these activities and to reflect carefully and critically about your ongoing progress as a nurse. Remember—nursing is a journey, not a destination.

We hope that you enjoy our book and that it helps you achieve success in your nursing journey. We'd be thrilled to hear what you think of the book and welcome suggestions for improvement. Please send your comments to <feedback@elsevier.com.au>.

Tracy Levett-Jones
Sharon Bourgeois

Chapter 1

The rules of engagement

Always bear in mind that your own resolution to succeed is more important than any one thing.

Abraham Lincoln (1809–65), 16th US president

Tips and tales 1.1
Know the lie of the land

The healthcare context has become increasingly complex, technological, consumer orientated and litigious over the last 20 years. Factors such as high patient throughput, increased acuity and decreased length of stay mean that hospitalised patients are sicker than ever before and stay in hospital for increasingly shorter periods of time. 'People now in general wards were in intensive care fifteen years ago, many people cared for in hospital are now cared for in the community, and the people who are now in intensive care would have died fifteen years ago' (Johnson & Preston 2001 p 6). These factors, coupled with current nursing shortages, have made nurses' working lives challenging, intense and often stressful. In fact, the clinical learning environment may resemble a 'minefield for the unwary'.

Something to think about...

It was the best of times; it was the worst of times.
Charles Dickens (1812–70), *A Tale of Two Cities*

Coaching tips

Why are we sharing this somewhat bleak outlook with you? Certainly not to discourage you from your chosen career path, but with the wisdom of knowing that 'forewarned is forearmed'. You'd be foolish to travel to a foreign land plagued by political and civil unrest without some degree of preparation in order to develop an understanding of the culture, people and context. The clinical learning environment is no different. Without an understanding of all that nursing in contemporary healthcare contexts means, you may well find yourself disillusioned by the dichotomy between what you *think* nurses and nursing should be and what they *actually* are.

Let's be very clear about one thing at this point, while the challenges associated with nursing in contemporary practice environments have escalated, the rewards, the satisfaction and the sheer joy in knowing you have made a difference are as wonderful today as they have always been. You will be inspired as you observe committed nurses providing extraordinary care despite, and perhaps even because of, the clinical challenges they encounter. Your mission (should you choose to accept it) is to navigate your way through what may seem at times to be a maze. This book will prepare you for your journey into this dynamic, exciting and challenging clinical environment.

Something to think about...

Travel plans are like honey, dripping down toward your lips—sweet anticipation.
Kurt Vonnegut (1922–), US novelist

Tips and tales 1.2
The clinical placement—what it is and why it matters

Clinical placements (sometimes called clinical practicum or fieldwork experiences) are where the world of nursing comes alive. At university/college you will learn *about nursing*. On your clinical placements you will learn *to nurse*. You will learn how nurses think, feel and behave, what they value and how they communicate. You will come to understand the culture and ethos of nursing in contemporary practice, as well as the problems, complexities and challenges nurses encounter. Some students say that clinical placements change the way they view the world. Whether this is true for you will depend to a large extent on how you approach it. Most importantly, clinical placements provide opportunities to engage with and care for clients, to enter their world, and to establish meaningful therapeutic relationships.

Clinical learning

Good nurses have a significant impact upon the clients and communities they serve. There is solid evidence (Aitken & Patrician 2000) that demonstrates that quality nursing care results in reductions in patient mortality and critical incidents such as medication errors, patient falls, hospital-acquired infections and pressure ulcers, to name a few. Clinical placements are where you apply the theory and knowledge gained through your academic pursuits to the reality of practice. Additionally, your clinical placement experiences will make explicit the areas in which you need more knowledge and experience. In this way knowledge pursuit and clinical application become an ongoing cycle of learning (Figure 1.1).

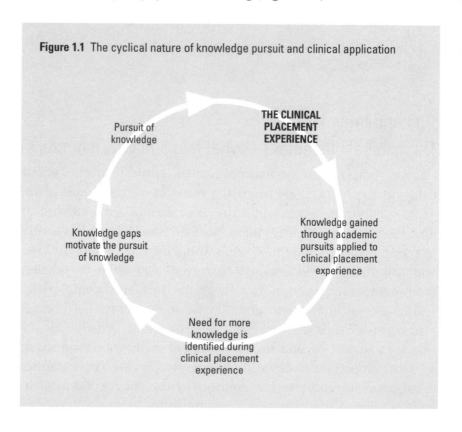

Figure 1.1 The cyclical nature of knowledge pursuit and clinical application

Pursuit of knowledge

THE CLINICAL PLACEMENT EXPERIENCE

Knowledge gaps motivate the pursuit of knowledge

Knowledge gained through academic pursuits applied to clinical placement experience

Need for more knowledge is identified during clinical placement experience

Clinical placement patterns

Depending on where you study, your clinical placement pattern will vary. Your placements may be scheduled in a 'block' pattern, in which you attend for a week or longer at a time, you may attend on regular days each week, or you may have a combination of both attendance patterns.

Clinical placement practice settings

Clinical placements occur across a broad range of practice settings and vary depending on where you study. Each clinical area has inherent learning opportunities and challenges. Typically you can expect to undertake placements in some or all of these areas:

- medical/surgical
- critical care
- older person care
- mental health
- community health
- maternal and child health
- disability services
- indigenous health
- rural and remote
- public and private health facilities

In Chapter 6 nursing experts from these practice areas share their insights. They provide an overview of each area, the unique learning opportunities available and the clinical challenges that you may encounter.

Clinical supervision and support

Various models of supporting and teaching students are used during clinical placements. The model implemented depends upon various factors, such as the context, the number of students and the student's level of experience.

You may have a clinical educator (sometimes called a facilitator) to guide your learning and to support you, or you may have a 'mentored' or 'preceptored' placement, in which you are guided by a clinician from the venue where you undertake your placement. Either way, it is important to remember that to a large extent the success of your placement will depend on what you bring to it and your degree of preparation and motivation.

Your feelings before, during and after your clinical placement experience will vary. Students report experiencing some or all of the following emotions: excitement, exhilaration, pride, confusion, anxiety, fear, apprehension, tension and stress. Your educator or mentor (or both) is there to support you. It is important to share your feelings and to seek further guidance and support whenever necessary.

Coaching tips

- The first step in preparing for your journey into the clinical placement is to make sure you are familiar with your educational institution's guidelines, procedures, policies and contact people.
- The second step (of course) is to read this book!

What's in a name?

When describing the people nurses care for, this book is peppered with the terms patient, client, healthcare consumer and resident. We made the decision to use these different terms deliberately. When you undertake clinical placements you'll quickly become aware that different terms are used to refer to those you care for, depending on the context of practice. We define the terms here so that you'll have a clear understanding of their meaning.

Patient is still the most common term used to describe a person seeking or receiving healthcare. It does carry some negative connotations, however, as traditionally a 'patient' was defined as someone who passively endured pain or illness. Although patients are becoming more active and proactive where their health is concerned, the term 'patient' is still the one you'll hear most often.

Client refers to the recipient of nursing care. 'Client' is a term that is inclusive of individuals, significant others, families and communities. It applies to people who are well and those who are experiencing health changes. It is intended to recognise the recipient of care as an active partner in that care and the need for the nurse to engage in professional behaviours that facilitate this active partnership. The term 'client' is often used in mental health and community health services.

Resident most often refers to a person who resides in a high- or low-care aged care facility or a person with a developmental disability who lives in a residential care facility, either short or long term.

Healthcare consumer is considered by some to be a politically correct term, particularly in the age of consumerism. Some writers (Sharkey 2003) suggest that the terms patient and client deny the health services user the rightful participation that is now expected in the Australian healthcare system. These

What's in a name? *(continued)*

commentators advocate that the term 'consumer' denotes a more active role in the planning and delivery of health services. In the 1990s the term 'consumer' became more common, particularly in mental health. It is important to note, however, that many writers deliberately avoid the use of the word 'consumer' when describing the people nurses care for, claiming that consumer is a negative and rather narrow definition of human beings in relationship to sickness and health.

As you can see there are divided opinions about the 'correct' terms to describe those we care for. We suggest that you keep an open mind during your clinical placements.

Tips and tales 1.3
Patient-centred care

'Patient- or person-centred care' is a term that has become prevalent in the nursing literature over the last decade. It is a notion that nurses hold dear, particularly in the increasingly complex and busy environments typical of contemporary practice. You will hear this term used frequently, so it is important to understand its meaning.

Patient- or person-centred care has been defined by McCormack (2004) as being concerned with the authenticity of the individual, that is, their personhood. It is a way of working that focuses on patients' personal beliefs, values, wants, needs and desires. Person-centred practice requires nurses to know the values held by their patients in order to treat them as individuals. Patient-centred care adopts approaches that enable flexibility, mutuality, respect, care and being with another in an interconnected relationship (McCormack 2001). Within this approach nurses must recognise patients' freedom to make their own decisions as a fundamental and valuable human right. Simply stated, patient-centred care means holistic care and placing people at the centre of all of the care decisions that are made.

Coaching tips

Consider the following situations.

A nurse was practising her intravenous cannulation skills, as she required 10 successful attempts to be re-accredited. Her patient, a 96-year-old woman, was admitted from an aged care facility with anaemia, secondary to a long history of melaena. The patient had expressed reluctance to have the blood transfusion that had been ordered for her. Despite the patient's obvious pain and distress, the nurse unsuccessfully attempted the cannulation four times, before giving up. She was dismissive of the patient's concerns about the transfusion.

Although it was important for this nurse to be re-accredited, was it more important than the patient's wellbeing? Was her care patient-centred? In the competing priorities evident in this scenario, did the patient's needs and values take precedence?

In another situation, a student nurse wanted to learn how to perform a urinary catheterisation. She entered the patient's room, explained that she was there to observe the catheterisation, and proceeded to watch the registered nurse perform the procedure. She did not seek the patient's consent nor was she aware of his discomfort and embarrassment resulting from her presence.

Once again the patient's feelings, needs and rights were not paramount. Even if the patient's verbal consent had been sought, the nurse should have paid careful attention to his non-verbal responses, such as facial expressions and body language that may well have revealed a different story.

We've given two examples where patient-centred care was not evident. Now we share a story where the opposite was true.

Emma [pseudonym] was an 18-year-old girl admitted to a palliative care unit with terminal cancer. All the nursing staff on the unit had become involved in her care, particularly the nurse unit manager. When Emma realised that she would not be returning home, she became terribly despondent. The manager spoke to her family and organised a secret 'rendezvous' in the hospital basement, at the service entrance. When Emma was wheeled down to the basement in her hospital bed, surrounded by infusion pumps, syringe drivers and other nursing paraphernalia, she was greeted by her adored Maltese terrier, Zoe. The look of absolute joy on Emma's face as Zoe snuggled into her arms for the last time was unforgettable.

This caring manager's organisation of a 'rendezvous' was a challenging feat, and one that probably contravened quite a few hospital rules, but it exemplifies perfectly what patient-centred care really means.

How nurses think, behave and speak should be underpinned by a commitment to patient-centred care. When caring for your patients reflect on whether your practice is patient-centred—our patients deserve nothing less.

Tips and tales 1.4
Models of care

Undertaking clinical placements in different facilities and units will provide you with exposure to different models of patient care. A model of care provides a framework for the way that patient care is organised within a clinical unit and relates to the way that nurses and other healthcare workers within the team structure patient-care activities. Differences in the models of care implemented within units or wards can be attributed to several factors, including the current worldwide shortage of nurses (Fagin 2001) and differences in skill mix (numbers, types and levels of experience of nurses and healthcare workers) (Davidson et al 2006; NSW Department of Health 2006; Viens et al 2005).

Models of patient care may include (NSW Department of Health 2006):

- task-oriented nursing
- team nursing
- patient allocation or total patient care, primary nursing or case management

Task-oriented nursing refers to a model where nurses undertake specific tasks related to nursing care across a group of patients. Some examples of task allocation may be when a nurse undertakes to shower all patients in a ward; another nurse may undertake the medications for the same group of patients. In this model of care delivery, nursing care relates to sets of activities that are performed by nurses for patients.

Team nursing is a model that 'teams' experienced permanent nurses with less experienced or casual staff to achieve nursing goals using a group approach. The size and skill mix of teams can vary from unit to unit and across healthcare facilities.

Patient allocation models were developed because nurses recognised the need for total patient care. The implementation of these types of models results in nurses getting to know the whole patient, rather than patients being cared for as a series of tasks. A nurse will be allocated to his or her patients (the number is dependent on factors such as patient need, staff mix and ward policies) and undertake all nursing care for the allocated patient/s (NSW Department of Health 2006).

The model of care delivery implemented on a ward will depend on a range of factors, including the degree of innovation and commitment by the people involved. Some models work better when there are sufficient numbers of highly qualified staff (RNs) to deliver care; others may focus on supporting less experienced staff using a team approach (NSW Department of Health 2006).

Activity

On your next placement, identify the model of care delivery used in the unit. Discuss with the nurses the reasons for the implementation of this model and its advantages and disadvantages. Find out where student nurses fit into this model.

Tips and tales 1.5
Competent practice

Competence is a complex concept that is difficult to define and measure (FitzGerald et al 2001). Many people make the mistake of thinking that competence simply means the satisfactory performance of a set task, but competence is so much more than this. Girot (1993, p 85) provides a more complete definition by suggesting that competence is 'the ability to combine knowledge, skills, behaviours, attitudes, values and beliefs appropriate to professional service delivery across a variety of contexts'.

The Australian Nursing and Midwifery Council (ANMC 2005) developed the National Competency Standards for the Registered Nurse to describe the attributes and performance required of a competent nurse in the clinical setting. The competency standards provide a benchmark for assessing competence. You will need to become very familiar with these standards, as your clinical performance will be assessed using these criteria and your eligibility for registration as a nurse will depend upon your demonstration of competence.

Keep in mind that 'competent' does not mean 'expert'. There are various levels of competence, but each of these has a minimum acceptable level or standard. Beginners are rarely expert, but they can be competent at performing a wide range of nursing activities methodically and well. They may be slow, but in time beginners develop organisational and time-management skills. They ask many questions (as they should), but they know the right questions to ask.

What does it all mean?

Competence. The combination of knowledge, skills, behaviours, attitudes, values and abilities that underpin effective and/or superior performance in a professional/occupational area.

Competent. The person has competence across all the domains of the competencies applicable to the nurses, at a standard that is judged to be appropriate for the level of the nurse being assessed.

Competency standards. These consist of ANMC competency units and competency elements (ANMC 2005).

Coaching tips

Recent reports from the National Review of Nursing Education (Heath et al 2002) and concerns expressed by nursing regulatory authorities (Nurses and Midwives Board of New South Wales 2005) highlight problems related to the development and demonstration of clinical competence by beginning nurses. In these coaching tips we suggest ways of developing your competence during your studies and throughout your nursing career.

Be knowledgable

- Focus on understanding the concepts and principles that underpin nursing care. Knowing why is just as important as knowing how.

- Ask questions, read widely, think carefully.
- Develop your library skills so that you can find the best information fast.
- Develop your research skills so that you can discern what is good, better and the best evidence for practice.
- When on a clinical placement, attend in-services whenever you have the opportunity.
- Find out when conferences are being held that are relevant to your learning and attend if possible—they are a great way of networking and accessing cutting-edge information.
- Aim high in your academic pursuits—don't be content with 'just a pass'.
- Attend all your lectures and tutorials on campus (don't skip classes).
- Commit to becoming a self-directed, lifelong learner. Remember, 'Knowledge keeps no better than fish' (Burnard & Chapman 1990, p 11) and given the rapid scientific and technological advances in the healthcare field, the knowledge gained in your program of study may soon become obsolete.

Develop your skills

- Work hard to develop your skills—attend all clinical skills sessions and actively participate.
- Don't miss an opportunity to practise. Many educational institutions encourage students to practise outside scheduled classes. These are valuable opportunities to consolidate your skills and identify any weaknesses.
- Observe expert clinicians caring for their patients. Ask them to supervise and critique your practice.
- There are many types of clinical skill checklists available and they are excellent for assessment purposes. Students can peer-review each other and your clinical educator may use them to assess you as well. In some programs the assessment

of core skills using a designated checklist is a compulsory
requirement.

- Tollefson's *Clinical psychomotor skills: assessment tools for
  nursing students* (2004) is an excellent text that contains a
  range of checklists and the related theoretical underpinnings.
  It is well worth a read.
- Continually ask yourself, 'is my practice safe and effective,
  and am I adhering to the principles of best practice?'

Reflect on your behaviours, values, attitudes and beliefs

- Nursing is a process of personal and professional growth.
  Throughout your studies, and indeed your career, it is vitally
  important to consider and reconsider your values, attitudes
  and beliefs continually, and to analyse how these attributes
  are reflected in your behaviours.
- Reflect on what it is that you value most—in yourself
  and in other professionals. Is it honesty, integrity, work
  ethic, compassion? Then consider how these values can be
  developed and integrated into your practice.
- Challenge your preconceptions. Listen and be open to
  other people's perspectives, particularly if their opinions are
  different from yours.
- Immerse yourself in a wide range of literature and media that
  challenge your thinking and the way you view the world.
- There are few worse criticisms for a nurse than to be called
  narrow-minded or bigoted.
- Embrace cultural diversity and open your mind (and heart)
  to people with different ethnicity, nationality, religion,
  language, age, gender and lifestyle—listen and learn!

Tips and tales 1.6
Working within your scope of practice

'Scope of practice' is a common term used extensively in nursing and other literature. However, the concept is not always clearly defined. In this section we define a nursing student's scope of practice as 'those nursing activities students are educated, competent and authorised to perform'. Nursing programs differ significantly, so students' scopes of practice will vary depending on where they are enrolled. Your scope of practice will develop as you progress through your nursing program and as your level of competence increases, and may vary depending on the context of your placement.

Why is it essential to understand and work within your scope of practice?

A scope of practice framework provides parameters that guide clinical learning and the nursing activities that you can participate in. It is not meant to unnecessarily limit your learning, but provides a clear outline of the types of activities that you should focus on. Consider the following situations.

A first-year student was concerned and upset about his unsatisfactory clinical appraisal. He felt discouraged because he was a high-achieving student who expected to receive an excellent appraisal. The educator had written the following comment: 'Ahmed is a hardworking and committed student but needs to work within his scope of practice and focus on consolidating skills appropriate to his level of enrolment'.

Ahmed was asked to describe his clinical placement and what had prompted this comment from the educator. Ahmed explained that he'd had a great placement, as he had been given wonderful learning opportunities by the registered nurses on his ward. He'd been permitted to do central line dressings, titrate intravenous (IV) infusions, manage patient-controlled analgesia (PCA), and more. He was proud that he had learnt skills well beyond those of most first-year students and was annoyed that the educator did not applaud his initiative.

Ahmed had focused on advanced and complex skills without having the necessary theoretical background. Ahmed had not learnt about central lines, infusion pumps, or patient-controlled analgesia at university and had little understanding of their purpose or potential complications. More worrying still was that Ahmed had been so focused on these advanced skills that he'd had little time to practise and consolidate the skills appropriate to his level of enrolment. He was not confident with patient hygiene nor was he able to administer oral medications safely. Ahmed was trying to run before he could walk.

Ahmed had practised nursing skills outside of his scope of practice and therefore was unsafe. This resulted in a failed grade for his clinical placement. While a scope of practice is not meant to limit learning opportunities, it provides a clear and structured framework for practice. It is sequentially developed, so that each new skill is related to and builds on those previously learnt. Most importantly, a scope of practice is supported by related theory.

Why do you need to discuss your scope of practice with the nurses you work with?

Clinicians frequently express the concern that they are not clear about what students have learnt on campus and in previous clinical placements. Additionally they are unsure of what clinical activities students are permitted to do and should be encouraged to engage in during clinical placements. Clinicians often describe instances where students attempt procedural skills beyond their level of ability or alternatively are reluctant to engage in clinical experiences outside of their 'comfort zone'. A clear outline of a student's scope of practice specific to each year of the program allows clinicians to support and challenge students based upon a collaborative understanding of expectations.

Coaching tips

- Make sure you access and understand the scope of practice appropriate to your university and year of enrolment.
- Clarify how your university requires the scope of practice to be used. Some educational institutions will not permit you to attempt any nursing procedures (a) that are not listed on the scope of practice document, (b) that you have not practised or (c) in which you have not demonstrated competency. Not all programs have the same requirements.
- Share your scope of practice with the nurses you work with, so that they know how they can best support and guide you.
- Use your scope of practice if you feel pressured to engage in nursing activities that are beyond your level of experience. Simply explain that your institution has parameters that guide your clinical learning. Of course you'll express your interest and say that you'd really like to watch the procedure being performed by an expert nurse.

Tips and tales 1.7
Clinical placements at distant locations

If you have the opportunity to undertake a clinical placement in another health service, state or country you are very fortunate. There is nothing like this type of experience to open your eyes to new possibilities. However, preparing for a clinical placement at a distance from where you live or study can be very daunting. Just like any other trip, you'll have travel and accommodation details to organise, as well as a host of other practical issues to sort out. On top of this there may be social and cultural differences between you, your co-workers and your clients to consider. Undoubtedly policies and procedures will be different from those you are used to and you won't have the immediate back-up of academic staff.

As if negotiating these issues isn't enough, you need to consider the learning opportunities available and your specific clinical objectives.

Undertaking a clinical placement at a distance can produce a lot of anxiety and this can impact on your learning and your ability to make the most of your experience. We outline here some strategies to help you through what can be a challenging time.

Coaching tips

Preparation

- Think about the type of placement that would suit you best, that you can afford and that you are passionate about. It's no good planning a placement with the Royal Flying Doctor Service if you hate flying!
- Distant placements can be expensive—look at all types of travel and accommodation options. Sharing expenses with fellow students may be possible. Investigate whether your educational institution, state or territory department of health or nursing organisations provide any financial support.
- Don't leave it to the last minute to get organised. This type of placement can take months to organise.
- Preparation requires research. Search on the intranet and internet and ask at travel agencies. Most importantly, talk to lecturers and students who have been to the placement institution. Ask lots of questions to get a realistic picture of what to expect.
- You'll need to know about accommodation options, parking, internet and library facilities, what to wear, who your contact person will be, what area you'll be working in, what they expect of you, what you'll be allowed to do.
- Make sure that you have a clear set of learning objectives (see section 3.12 for more information about clinical objectives).

When you arrive

- Be positive and enthusiastic. Let the people you work with know that you are excited to be there, ready to work and anxious to learn.
- Define your student role—in some places you may be expected to just 'tag along', in others to work as part of the team.
- Make sure that you discuss your expectations and learning objectives early in the placement.
- Be open to and welcoming of serendipitous learning opportunities.
- Keep a journal—write down the things you encounter and your reactions to it all. It will help you maintain perspective and will be great to look back on.
- Maintain regular contact with your academic support person. Keep the dialogue open and don't be afraid to ask lots of questions. If you are finding it difficult to meet your learning objectives, discuss this early so that an alternative leaning plan can be organised.
- Know when and where to seek help and don't hesitate to do so.
- Work to resolve conflict (for strategies, see section 3.4).
- Be prepared for things to go wrong. It is unusual for clinical placements to proceed without a hitch. Laugh; keep your sense of humour. Try to see something of value in each new problem and challenge.

Tips and tales 1.8
Who shall I turn to?

Different models of clinical support and teaching are used during clinical placements. The model selected depends upon factors such as clinical context, the numbers of students on placement and their level of experience.

Most educational institutions employ clinical educators, sometimes called facilitators, to support, teach and assess groups of students. In addition to, or sometimes instead of, clinical educators, you'll often be teamed up with a registered nurse when on a clinical placement. Depending on the organisational structure of the unit and its staffing levels, you may work with the same registered nurse for the whole time you are on the placement or alternatively you may work with a different nurse every day. There are some advantages to both models. Working with the same nurse provides a measure of security and continuity, but you are exposed to only one way of doing things. When you work with different nurses you'll experience a range of different practices and ways of nursing and this will help clarify the type of nurse you want to be.

In Australia the terms *mentoring* and *preceptoring* have evolved and are often used interchangeably to describe a supportive educative role. Mentorship and preceptorship have been described as the most common forms of clinical supervision and support. Both types of supportive relationships have the potential to ease the transition between the relatively sheltered world of academia and the health-service environment, with all its contemporary challenges and pressures.

Coaching tips

Irrespective of whether you are supported by a mentor, preceptor, buddy, practice partner or clinical educator, to a large extent the success of the relationship will depend on you. You need to be very clear of your learning objectives (see section 3.12), as these will frame your learning, and you must be able to explain and elaborate on them so that the person you are working with can support you and guide you towards achieving them. Occasionally your support person may suggest that your objectives need to be modified or

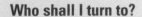

Who shall I turn to?

Mentor Traditionally mentoring referred to a mutual and committed relationship between a student or new employee and an experienced staff member. The relationship developed over time and created opportunities for students or new employees to gain valuable skills and knowledge, to become socialised and acculturated to the organisation and its ways of operating, and to become proficient in the new role under the direct guidance of the mentor.

Preceptor Traditionally preceptoring referred to an orientation technique, where qualified staff were formally assigned to orientate students or new employees to a designated area over short periods of time. The preceptor acted as a role model and resource person, helping with the process of socialisation.

Buddy The forces in contemporary practice, such as staffing shortages and increased casualisation of the workforce, sometimes work against sustaining the ongoing supportive relationships of mentoring and preceptoring. A buddy is a term that has come to mean a nurse that you work with on a day-to-day basis and not necessarily on an ongoing basis.

Practice partner This more contemporary term refers to a nurse that you work with, often in the final year or semester of your nursing program, who guides and supports you to become increasingly independent, competent, autonomous and responsible.

Clinical educators/facilitators These may be employed on a casual basis or seconded from the clinical facilities. Clinical educators assist and enable students in a clinical setting to acquire the required knowledge, skills and attitudes to meet the standards defined by the university and nurse regulatory authorities. Clinical educators liaise between students and academic and clinical staff in a tripartite relationship and are responsible for supporting, teaching and assessing groups of students, often across different wards or units.

Based on Andrews & Roberts 2003; Clare et al 2003; Clare et al 2002; Hughes 2002 amended if they are not achievable or appropriate for a particular environment.

You need to be able to define your scope of practice so that your support person is aware of what you can and can't do. You will probably find that this person will observe and assess you for a while before entrusting you with patient care. Don't take this personally or as an indication of a lack of confidence in your ability. It is only to be expected, because registered nurses maintain responsibility for their patients at all times and your support person needs to be very sure of your abilities before allowing you to practise with any measure of independence.

If a situation arises in which you feel that your relationship with your support person is not working, try resolving it with him or her in the first instance. Be open to his or her viewpoints, as it may just be a problem of miscommunication. However, if this does not improve the situation or if you feel uncomfortable about trying to resolve it, you should seek the support and guidance of someone experienced who you feel you can trust to handle the situation professionally—your academic support person may be ideal.

Nursing mirrors what happens in everyday life and sometimes personality clashes arise. Hopefully these can be managed in a positive, professional and constructive manner, but at times it may be best for you to work with a different person.

Be mindful that experiencing a series of personality clashes may indicate that you need some guidance in managing interpersonal relationships.

Something to think about...

Mentors remind us that we can indeed survive the terror of the coming journey and undergo the transformation by moving through, not around our fear. Mentors give us the magic that allows us to enter the darkness, a talisman to protect us from evil spells, a gem of wise advice, a map, and sometimes simply courage. But always the mentor appears near the onset of the journey as a helper, equipping us in some way for what is to come, a midwife to our dreams, a 'keeper of the promise'. Success is a lot slipperier without a mentor to show us the ropes. The mentor is clearly concerned with the transmission of wisdom. They do this by leading us on the journey of our lives. We trust them because they have been there before. They embody our hopes, cast light on the way ahead, interpret arcane signs, warn us of lurking dangers, and point out unexpected delights along the way.

Daloz 1999, Parkes 1986

Tips and tales 1.9
Working hard—but not too hard

Nursing students frequently express how important it is for them to fit in—to belong and be accepted as part of the nursing team. This is not surprising given that the need to belong has been cited as a fundamental human need (Baumeister & Leary 1995; Maslow 1987). Students who try too hard to fit in sometimes sacrifice their 'student status' to become one of the 'workers'. It is not unusual for students, believing that their hard work will help them to be valued as part of the team, to fill their clinical placement days with a series of disjointed nursing tasks (making beds, taking vital signs, bathing patients) rather than developing their ability to nurse holistically across a range of areas. Don't be confused! We are not saying that undergraduate students are above basic nursing skills. On the contrary, we are saying that as a student you need to be proactive in identifying and maximising valuable learning opportunities across a range of areas and at different levels.

Something to think about...

When a child stands in awe of the mystery of a falling rose petal, then it's time to teach the law of gravity.
Anonymous

Coaching tips

Give yourself permission to be a student! Articulate your learning objectives and assessment requirements. Be on the look out for serendipitous learning opportunities. Listen closely in handover and relate your clinical objectives to the clinical issues identified. Did someone mention a complex diabetic leg ulcer that needs to be re-dressed? Do you have wound management as one of your objectives? Take the initiative. Ask if you can watch the wound dressing being performed, then go home that night and read all you can about diabetic ulcers. The next day ask if you can undertake the procedure under supervision. As a student it is your responsibility to link theory and practice and you will have countless opportunities to do so (if you are on the lookout for them). Linking theory to practice will allow you to develop your repertoire of knowledge and skills in a way that is clinically relevant.

Ask if you can care for increasing numbers of patients (under supervision), so that you can develop your time-management and organisational skills (even in first year). Certainly, while caring for groups of patients you'll be doing so-called 'basic skills' (never forget how important they are and how much consolidation they need), but you'll also be extending your practice and learning to nurse holistically rather than in a task-oriented way.

Don't fool yourself into thinking that if you just 'get on with the job' you'll fit in and be accepted. You are much more likely to earn the respect of your colleagues by fully embracing your student status, asking questions, seeking out learning opportunities and showing an interest.

Tips and tales 1.10
Privacy

Government legislation requires the protection of personal information and the privacy of others. This type of legislation ensures that information about you as an individual is not used without your consent or for illegal purposes. Privacy is a right for all individuals and you will need to ensure that you understand your obligations in respect of privacy laws.

You are obliged to protect and maintain personal information about others during the course of clinical placement. Likewise you can also expect that your own personal information is protected. Personal information is information that can identify a person. This could include your name, address or phone number. In some circumstances it may be your DNA, fingerprints or body samples. Health information (for example, health records) is also protected (Privacy NSW 2004).

Information about individuals must not be used illegally or given to others without the individual's consent. Most educational institutions will have processes available for students to lodge concerns if they feel that their privacy has been breached. Health facilities also have these mechanisms available to patients and staff. You need to take care to ensure that you do not inadvertently disclose personal information. Some areas where you will need to be particularly mindful include the taking of notes during handover and any discussions you are involved in, including debriefing sessions.

Aside from considering patient privacy concerns, on clinical placements you will be exposed to issues that may affect other students. Be prudent in your behaviours, to ensure that circumstances on clinical placement for a fellow student are not relayed to other students on campus. The following story relates an example that occurred recently.

Mary was on the same ward as André for their second-year placement. Over the last few days, André had been arguing with his clinical educator about what he believed he should be doing. The clinical educator had pointed out that André was to care for his allocated patients to the level of his knowledge and was not on placement just to undertake clinical assessments. André was instructed to negotiate his learning with staff, as well as to take responsibility for the care of his patients. Over the course of the placement, several staff had complained to the clinical educator about André's lack of patient care. The clinical educator discussed the issues and strategies for improvement with André, but following a lack of improvement he eventually received an unsatisfactory grade for his clinical placement.

On return to university the following week, André was angry when several colleagues spoke to him about his unsatisfactory grade. While his name had not been disclosed, the circumstances surrounding the issues had allowed him to be recognised by other students on campus. André confronted Mary about how other students had become aware of his clinical result and her role in disclosing information about his placement.

In this scenario, Mary had revealed private information about André. While she had not mentioned his name, the other students were able to identify him. André's clinical placement results constitute personal information.

Remember, the privacy of individuals and personal information is protected by government legislation and in all situations you must protect the personal information of others.

Coaching tips

- Be aware of what constitutes privacy and breaches of privacy.
- Protect information about a person whose identity is apparent or whose identity can be reasonably ascertained from information provided.
- As a guiding principle, what occurs in an area or situation should remain with those involved and should not be discussed by others (i.e. avoid gossip).
- Access to any patient information, including patient notes, requires permission.
- Gain consent to use potentially identifiable information (written consent is preferable). Some circumstances may require the medical officer and the nursing unit manager to give consent.
- Remember that the right of individuals is to have control over any personal information and that others must obtain valid consent for the use of that information.
- Only collect the minimum amount of information about a person after obtaining their consent.
- Seek advice and guidance from management about policies and protocols in operation at every facility where you are placed. These will vary depending on the type of facility, its guiding policies and your health-department directives.

Tips and tales 1.11
Confidentiality

Something to think about...

Responsibility for sensitive confidential information about clients or patients is often both a burden and a privilege for carers, but it also gives them a special relationship with those in their care and subtle power over them.
Thompson et al 2000, p 119

Confidentiality can be defined as a professional obligation to respect privileged information between health provider and client. Consider the following situation.

Joseph was sitting on the ledge outside the coffee shop when his nursing student colleagues wandered over to join him. They were excited about having witnessed the birth of a baby and wanted to share their experiences. However, Joseph became uncomfortable when one of his colleagues began to speak explicitly about processes related to the delivery, complications that had occurred and even mentioned the name the parents had given their new baby. Joseph cautioned his colleagues about maintaining confidentiality and requested that they keep their voices low, so that people nearby could not hear. While his colleagues were initially annoyed about being criticised and felt somewhat belittled by Joseph's comments, they soon complied.

People often disclose sensitive and sometimes private information about themselves to health professionals. However, in doing so, patients make themselves vulnerable (Thompson 2000). Safeguards to protect this vulnerability of patients are nested within the concept of confidentiality. When information is required for quality improvement or research purposes, informed consent must be provided and the anonymity of patients protected.

Confidentiality is a broad concept that extends the concept of privacy. Although nurses may discuss personal details and care related to patients, this discussion should be constrained by ethical standards and responsible judgment. The Code of Professional Conduct for Nurses in Australia determines that nurses must treat as confidential personal information obtained in a professional capacity (ANMC 2003).

Coaching tips

- Do not use patient experiences as 'conversation pieces'. Disclosing bits of information may assist a listener to identify a person, place or set of processes and therefore breaches confidentiality. Confidentiality means that you need to consider how information is used, handled, stored or restricted.
- Be aware of how you document handover notes and how these are used and safeguarded throughout your shift and following your shift.
- Ensure that you are familiar with policies and protocols in operation at healthcare facilities. These vary according to the type of facility and governmental policies and include data used for assignment preparation. Use of client's notes and photographs will need to comply with the facility's protocols.

Tips and tales 1.12
First impressions last

It's a sad but true fact that first impressions are formed within seconds of meeting and those impressions are based most often on appearance. Forget what you see on television. In the real world of nursing, a very specific dress code exists. The clinical environment is focused on safety—yours and that of the patients—and this to a large extent dictates what is considered acceptable in appearances in general, and uniforms in particular.

Don't be caught unaware— before you start your placement, check your educational institution's requirements as well as those of your placement venue. Some placements have special requirements—for example, mental health facilities may prefer smart casual clothes, while operating theatres usually provide surgical attire.

Below we offer some guidelines based on our experiences of what most clinical venues expect. We tried to find a way of writing this section that was discreet and delicate, but eventually decided to just 'say it like it is'!

Coaching tips

- Uniforms should be neat, complete, comfortable, correctly fitting, clean and wrinkle-free.
- Shoes must be comfortable (for obvious reasons) and comply with occupational health and safety standards (non-slip, fully enclosed, leather). Runners are great for sport but not for a clinical placement.
- Heavy makeup is not appropriate for clinical placement—it is best left for your leisure time. Overpowering perfumes should be avoided, as they can cause patients to become nauseated.
- Nails should be clean, short, filed and without nail polish for infection control purposes. It is easy to tear the fragile skins of elderly patients or penetrate gloves with long or sharp nails. Chipped nail polish and artificial nails have been shown to harbour infectious microorganisms.
- Long hair must be clean and tied back firmly.
- Leave your jewellery at home. Wristwatches are problematic as they can scratch patients and need to be removed each time you wash your hands. A fob watch with a second hand is more convenient. Similarly, rings can scratch patients and cause cross-infection. A plain band is usually acceptable in most clinical areas. One pair of small studs (in ears only) may be accepted, but bracelet/s or necklace/s are not to be worn (unless of the medic alert type). Many a confused person has pulled or grabbed at a dangling necklace or earring (ouch!).
- For those placements where smart casual clothing is requested in lieu of uniform, avoid wearing revealing clothing.

It may not be polite to mention the following issues in refined company but...

- Please shower/bath daily (and wear deodorant).
- There is nothing worse for a nauseated patient than being cared for by a nurse with bad breath. Clean teeth and fresh breath are essential.
- For men, beards should be neat and trimmed.
- Last but not least, make sure you always wear your ID or name badge and have your personal protective equipment (for example, safety glasses) with you on clinical placements.

Tips and tales 1.13
Competing needs

A supportive clinical learning environment is viewed as essential to maximising student readiness for practice (Clare et al 2003). The very nature of the clinical placement experience, however, can create competition between the educational needs of students and the service needs of the facility. Students enter an environment where financial constraints, technology, the pace of change and staff mix can impact on optimal clinical learning experiences.

Some clinical placements can create a situation where the fulfilment of your personal learning needs competes with service needs. An example would be when you are allocated a patient load but the needs of your allocated patients do not align with your clinical objectives. You may be required to care for patients with completely different conditions from those that you had hoped to focus on, and therefore your ability to meet your goals is substantially reduced. In another situation, the educational institution requirements may be incongruent with the clinical practice model implemented—for example, when the unit uses a model of team nursing and the student expects to care holistically for a group of patients.

Coaching tips

* Develop an understanding of the different clinical practice models used in the clinical environment.
* Negotiate your learning needs with your clinical educator and mentor early in the placement. Do not leave this to the last day.
* Openly discuss any concerns that you have with competing needs as soon as they become apparent and, with your mentor and clinical educator, identify strategies to address them.

Tips and tales 1.14
The generation gap

Sixty per cent of nurses in Australia are aged over 40 years. It is widely accepted that almost half of the current nursing workforce will contemplate retirement in the next 10–15 years. By 2010 Australia will need 10,000–13,000 new graduates each year to meet workforce needs (AHWAC 2004). This means that in the nursing profession there is, and will continue to be, a wide generational cross-section. So let's think about nursing generations, and where you fit in.

A generation is an aggregate of people who share birth years, a common location in history and a collective persona. In nursing there may be up to three generations of nurses working together in one clinical area. Each generation has its own set of expectations, values, goals and motivators, and it is almost inevitable that there will be some clashes due to a lack of mutual understanding. Below we describe some of the attributes of the different generations that you may encounter on a clinical placement.

Generational diversity

Baby boomers (born 1941–60)

Baby boomers comprise the largest generation and are said to be characterised by rebellion in their youth and conservatism in their thirties, forties and beyond. They share the common traits of ambition, loyalty and optimism. They are highly committed to their employer, often regarded as workaholics and reluctant to change jobs.

Generation X (born 1961–81)

While career advancement and personal development are key to this generation's happiness, they are constantly trying to balance career, family and leisure activities. They tend to be sceptical, competitive, autonomous, image conscious and in need of regular feedback about their performance. They value fun and humour in the workplace and are open to new job opportunities.

Generation Y (born 1981 onwards)

Members of this generation are highly aware of their rights and have a perception of workplace entitlements. They expect their employers to be flexible and to accommodate individual needs. They want to be continually learning and challenged, and are perceived to have short attention spans. They are conversant with technology. They are altruistic, ambitious and independent workers, who are socially and environmentally responsible. They see job and career change as inevitable. (Kupperschmidt 1998, 2001; Weston 2001)

What generation X thinks of baby boomers

- They are workaholics.
- They are self-righteous.
- They thrive on work-related politics.
- They demand constant validation.
- They need to lighten up—it's only a job!
- They are set in their ways.
- They have quit learning and are stuck in a rut—'this is the way we've always done it!'
- They are not technologically competent.
- They are cynical and pessimistic (I knew this would happen).
- They need to get along with people and be liked.

What baby boomers think of generation X

- They are lazy.
- They are wingers.
- They spend too much time on the internet and email.
- They are self-focused.
- They are demanding and refuse to wait their turn.
- They have no work ethic.
- They are not loyal.
- They don't show respect.
- They aren't committed.
- They have a 'you owe me' attitude.
- They are easily bored.

What generation X and baby boomers think of generation Y

- They are too competitive.
- They are more focused on learning and less on getting the work done.
- They are obsessed with information technology.
- They are aloof and tolerate teamwork only when absolutely necessary.
- They need supervision, guidance, support and mentoring.

(Based on Kupperschmidt 1998, 2001; Weston 2001)

Coaching tips

- Which generation do you belong to? Think about the extent to which the attributes described apply to you.
- Next time you undertake a clinical placement, consider the different generations that comprise the nursing team.
- Be aware that the different generational attitudes towards work, learning, technology, feedback and teamwork is likely to result in misunderstandings at times and try not to take it personally. Remember 'understanding breeds tolerance'.

Tips and tales 1.15
The roles and functions of the interdisciplinary healthcare team

Efficient workplace practices come about by understanding and appreciating the diverse skills and expertise of the different members of the interdisciplinary healthcare team.

Aside from nurses, the interdisciplinary healthcare team may include medical and allied health personnel, pharmacists, pathologists, psychologists, counsellors, radiologists, occupational therapists and speech pathologists, to name a few. Table 1.1 identifies some of the different people you may encounter on a clinical placement.

Table 1.1 People you may encounter on a clinical placement

Role	Definition
Students—nursing and midwifery	People who are enrolled in educational programs accredited by registration boards that authorise nursing. These may include undergraduate nurses, enrolled nurses and student midwives.
Registered nurse (RN)	A person whose name is entered on the register allocated to registered nurses (i.e. Division 1 or List A). Application to practise is renewed yearly with the authorising board in the state where practise is to be undertaken. Registered nurses are accountable for the provision of nursing care to a broad group of patients.
Enrolled nurse	A person whose name is entered on the register allocated to enrolled nurses (i.e. division 2 or list B). Application to practise is renewed yearly with the authorising board in the state where practice is to be undertaken. Enrolled nurses practise nursing under the direction of a registered nurse.
	An extension of the category of enrolled nurse (e.g. endorsed enrolled nurse) is the person who performs at an advanced level and is delegated higher responsibilities under the supervision of a registered nurse or midwife.

Continued

Table 1.1 People you may encounter on a clinical placement *(continued)*

Role	Definition
Midwife	A person whose name is entered in the register for practice (i.e. division 1 or list A). Application to practise is renewed yearly with the authorising board in the state where practice is to be undertaken. Qualifications and experience are approved by the registering authority, to render the person capable of providing maternity services to mothers and babies.
Nurse practitioner	A registered nurse and/or midwife who has been educated in an advanced clinical role and whose scope of practice is determined by his or her context of practice.
Healthcare workers	Various roles are undertaken by healthcare workers. They may function independently or in collaboration with the interdisciplinary healthcare team. An example would be the Aboriginal healthcare worker. Some roles may be accountable to the registered nurse or midwife.
Unregulated carers	A variety of roles exist for people to care for patients without licensing requirements. They may undertake activities delegated by the registered nurse or midwife according to their competence. Examples are carers, personal care assistants, assistants in nursing, Aboriginal healthcare workers etc.
Patient care attendants	People employed by a facility to support the care requirements of patients. They may have functions that involve moving or positioning patients and/or equipment, attending to personal needs of patients, or disposal of soiled equipment. Functions associated with this position are varied and often depend on the context of the area in which they are employed.
Technicians	Various technical positions abound in healthcare facilities. Some of these have replaced nursing roles and others have supplementary roles in the care of clients. Examples of technical staff are technicians who work with specialist equipment—for example, anaesthetic technicians and sterile-supply technicians.

Continued

Table 1.1 People you may encounter on a clinical placement *(continued)*

Role	Definition
Medical personnel	You will encounter several levels of medical personnel during placement. Public healthcare facilities employ resident medical officers, whereas other institutions may use the consultancy services of medical officers. This will depend on the nature of the facility (i.e. public or private) and the agreements in place between the facility and medical officer. Resident medical officers usually encountered in public hospitals include the following: • Intern • Resident medical officer (year 1–4) • Registrar (year 1–4) • Senior registrar Consultant medical officers may have the following positions: anaesthetists, surgeons, obstetricians, gynaecologists, physicians, pathologists, psychiatrists etc.
Psychologists	People who are engaged in the scientific study of the mind and behaviour, and may assist through clinical treatment and teaching. They may be concerned with different areas such as sport and exercise, education and occupational or clinical psychology.
Podiatrist	Practitioners of podiatry (chiropody) who deal with the treatment of feet and their ailments.
Occupational therapist	People who employ a form of therapy for those recuperating from physical or mental disease or injury. They encourage rehabilitation through performance of the activities of daily living (such as washing and dressing, hobbies, crafts etc).
Speech pathologists	People concerned with the study and treatment of clients with speech, communication, language and swallowing problems.
Counsellors	People who support clients to deal with personal problems that do not involve psychological disorders.

Based on Baron & Kalsher 2002; Concise Medical Dictionary (Oxford Reference Online); NSW Department of Health, 27 January 2005; Nurses and Midwives Board of New South Wales 2005; Nurses Board of Western Australia 2004

Coaching tips

- Attend interdisciplinary healthcare team meetings when possible.
- Become familiar with the roles and functions of all staff encountered on each clinical placement.
- Develop an understanding of how team members communicate and work collaboratively to provide quality care.

Tips and tales 1.16
Networking

Nursing is all about building and maintaining relationships—in business this is called networking. Clinical placements provide wonderful opportunities for students to meet new people and to develop strong networks. Nurturing professional relationships is a mechanism that students should develop during their course, as it has the potential to open many doors. Establishing your network is a powerful strategy to achieve career goals.

Networking is about capitalising on the multiple relationships that you'll develop as a student. The process begins by thinking of the people who share your interests and values and who could be helpful to you now and in the future: fellow students, academic staff, clinical experts, educators or managers, for example. The people you network with may be those from whom you need help or advice. They may also be those who require your help or advice. You may be surprised how far the 'ripples' of networking extend.

I remember Joaquin, a cleaner who worked on the first ward I worked on as a registered nurse. He was new to Australia, having recently migrated from South America. He was a tireless worker and always ready to help. He related well to staff and patients alike. As we were both new to the unit, a camaraderie developed between us. He was studying to become a nurse and I gave him some nursing texts. Our lives soon diverged but 17 years later I met Joachin again at an interview. He was then the manager of the unit to which I'd applied.

Coaching tips

- List the people in your current network, and then list the people you'd like to network with in the future. Think about the type of people that could help you achieve your career goals and those that may benefit from your help.
- Don't be afraid to ask for the help or advice you need (most people love to be needed).
- Reach out to others who may need your help and advice, such as new students and international students.
- If you meet a registered nurse who particularly inspires you, ask if she or he would agree to act as a professional mentor throughout your program.
- Apply for a position as an assistant in nursing to gain exposure to different people and opportunities.
- Ask if there is a mechanism for you to apply for employment on wards that you particularly enjoyed, or if you can return for another placement at a later date.
- Ask the manager and/or other staff members if they would act as referee(s) for you.
- Join professional nursing groups (many have student rates) to develop networks and relationships. These groups can provide opportunities for you to access mentors.
- Be open to the opportunities available for your graduate employment and make the most of the networking prospects.

Reflective thinking activities

Think about what motivated you to become a nurse and what you expected nursing to be like. Have your experiences been different from what you initially expected? In what ways have your nursing experiences exceeded your expectations? Are there any ways in which nursing has disappointed you?

How can you ensure that you achieve your learning objectives in clinical environments even when the staff are busy and the area is short-staffed?

What do you think are your most important rights and responsibilities as a nursing student?

References

AHWAC 2004 Nursing workforce planning in Australia—a guide to the process and methods used by the Australian Health Workforce Committee, Australian Health Workforce Advisory Committee Report, 2004. Online. Available <http://www.health.nsw.gov.au/amwac/projects.html>, 27 December 2005.

Aitken L & Patrician P 2000 Measuring organizational traits of hospitals: the revised nursing work index. Nursing Research 49(3):146–153.

Andrews M & Roberts D 2003 Supporting student nurses learning in and through clinical practice: the role of the clinical guide. Nurse Education Today 23:474–481.

ANMC 2003 Code of professional conduct for nurses in Australia. Australian Nursing and Midwifery Council, Dickson (ACT).

— 2005 ANMC National Competency Standards for the Registered Nurse. Australian Nursing and Midwifery Council, Canberra.

Baron R A & Kalsher M J 2002 Essentials of psychology. Allyn and Bacon, Boston.

Baumeister R & Leary M 1995 The need to belong: desire for interpersonal attachments as a fundamental human motivation. Psychological Bulletin 117(3):497–529.

Burnard P & Chapman C 1990 Nurse education: the way forward. Scutari Press, Middlesex, UK.

Clare J, Brown D, Edwards H et al 2003 Evaluating clinical learning environments: creating education–practice partnerships and clinical education benchmarks for nursing. Learning outcomes and curriculum development in major disciplines: nursing phase 2 final report, March. School of Nursing and Midwifery, Flinders University, Adelaide.

Clare J, White J, Edwards H et al 2002 Curriculum, clinical education, recruitment, transition and retention in nursing: final report for the AUTC, January. School of Nursing and Midwifery, Flinders University, Adelaide.

Daloz N 1999 Guiding the journey of adult learners. Jossey Bass, San Francisco.

Davidson P, Halcomb E, Hickman L et al 2006 Beyond rhetoric: what do we mean by a 'model of care'? Australian Journal of Advanced Nursing 23(3):47–55.

Fagin CM 2001 When care becomes a burden: diminishing access to adequate nursing. Online. Available <http://www.milbank.org/010216fagin.html>, 23 April 2001.

FitzGerald M, Walsh K & McCutcheon H 2001 An integrative systematic review of indicators for competence for practice and protocol for validation of indicators of competence. Conducted by the Joanna Briggs Institute for Evidence Based Nursing and Midwifery. Commissioned by the Queensland Nursing Council. Adelaide University, Adelaide.

Girot E 1993 Assessment of competence in clinical practice: a review of the literature. Nurse Education Today 13:83–90.

Heath P, Duncan P, Lowe E & Macri S 2002 National review of nursing education 2002—our duty of care. Department of Education, Science and Training (DEST), Canberra.

Hughes C 2002 Issues in supervisory facilitation. Studies in continuing education, 24(1):57–71.

Johnson D & Preston B 2001 Australia: an overview of issues in nursing education. Online. Available <http://www.detya.gov.au/highered/eippubs/eip01_12fullreport.htm>, 30 April 2005.

Kupperschmidt B 1998 Understanding generation X employees. Journal of Nursing Administration 28(12):36–43.

— 2001 Understanding next generation employees. Journal of Nursing Administration 31(12):570–574.

Maslow A 1987 Motivation and personality, 3rd edn. Harper and Row, New York.

McCormack B 2004 Person-centredness in gerontological nursing: an overview of the literature. International Journal of Older People Nursing 13(3a):31–38.

NSW Department of Health 2006 First report on the models of care project, February–April 2005. NSW Department of Health, North Sydney.

— 2005 Public hospital (medical officers) award—hours of work and tenure (27 January). Online. Available <www.health.nsw.gov.au/policies>, 7 February 2006.

Nurses and Midwives Board of New South Wales 2005 NMB guidelines for registered nurses and enrolled nurses regarding the boundaries of professional practice. Online. Available <www.nmb.nsw.gov.au/bounds/guidelin.htm>, 22 November 2005.

Nurses Board of Western Australia (2004) Scope of nursing practice decision-making framework. Online. Available <www.nbwa.org.au>, 13 January 2006.

Parkes S 1986 The critical years: the young adult's search for faith to live by. Harper, San Francisco.

Privacy NSW 2004 NSW privacy essentials. Office of the NSW Privacy Commissioner, Sydney South, 2 April, pp 1–8.

Sharkey R 2003 The relationship between nursing care and positive health outcomes for consumers with long term serious mental illness. PhD thesis, University of Newcastle, Newcastle.

Thompson I E, Melia KM & Boyd KM 2000 Nursing ethics. Churchill Livingstone, Edinburgh.

Tollefson J 2004 Clinical psychomotor skills: assessment tools for nursing students, 2nd edn. Social Science Press, Tuggerah.

Viens C, Lavoie-Tremblay M, Leclerc MM & Brabant LH 2005 New approaches to organizing care and work. The Health Care Manager 24(2):150–158.

Weston M 2001 Coaching generations in the workplace. Nursing Administration Quarterly 25(2):11–21.

Chapter 2

Great expectations

That was a memorable day to me, for it made great changes in me. Pause you who read this, and think for a moment...on one memorable day...

Charles Dickens (1812–70), *Great Expectations*

Tips and tales 2.1
Patients' expectations

What do patients expect from their nurse? This should be a very easy question to answer. Ask your friends, family and fellow students this question and you are bound to get a wide range of responses. What nursing attributes do you think are most important to patients?

We know from a variety of studies over the last 15 years that the skills of caring, empathy, listening, 'being with', comforting, intuiting, assessment, planning and communication are the qualities that patients value most highly (McCormack et al 1999). However, the saying 'the patient doesn't care how much you know, the patient wants to know how much you care' is not always true. Certainly patients want to be able to depend on you to take care of them with kindness and empathy, but with the increasingly complex world of healthcare, patients want to be sure that you know what you are doing and why.

So what does this mean for students? If patients expect to be cared for by nurses with expertise and experience how do students gain opportunities to learn and practise? You'll be relieved to know that on the whole patients are very tolerant of students. If you fumble the first few times when taking a temperature or blood pressure, patients will usually understand. When you are slow at doing a dressing or removing an IV, they'll make allowances because you are still learning. Patients will not expect you to be able to answer all their questions, but they will expect you to find someone who can.

There are some things that patients do not make allowances for, irrespective of the nurse's experience or level. Patients expect a student nurse to be as respectful of their privacy as any other nurse. They expect you to be honest about what you know and don't know, and can and can't do. They expect you to be courteous and to treat them with dignity at all times. Even though you are a learner, patients still expect you to carry out procedures safely and accurately and to acknowledge your limitations.

Patients often comment that they appreciate being cared for by students, because they take the time to stop and talk. In busy hospital units this is often undervalued. Many patients also like to feel that they have been involved in the clinical education of student nurses and will happily explain their history, diagnosis, treatment regimen and medications. Listen carefully; without doubt, you will learn a great deal from your patients—they are the experts about their lives and health conditions. Listen to them, learn from them and appreciate their stories. They contain a wealth of information.

Coaching tips

- Make sure you are prepared before you enter a patient's room. It is very disconcerting for a patient when a student has no idea of what they are doing, or why. If you are giving a subcutaneous injection, for example, review the procedure; discuss the details with your mentor, and ask as many questions as necessary, before you approach your patient.
- Admit when you are out of your depth. If an infusion pump is alarming and you don't know how to deal with it, don't stand there for 5 minutes hoping you'll get a moment of inspiration. Find someone who can assist you (then watch and learn).
- If you are taking a blood pressure or any other observation, and you are really not sure if your result is correct, be honest and ask someone to check it for you.
- Remember that, while technical competence is essential, nursing should not be reduced to a series of tasks lacking the therapeutic qualities that are so important to patients.

Tips and tales 2.2
Clinicians' expectations

Over the years we have found that clinicians have the following expectations of nursing students undertaking a clinical placement. Take some time to think about each of these points. Students should:

- understand the nursing context and work they are involved in.
- know when to ask for help.
- know where to go for help.
- recognise their own limitations and deficits.
- demonstrate commitment to the nursing team.
- ask questions and question practice.
- be critically thinking problem-solvers.
- be enthusiastic, motivated, positive and excited to be a nurse on a clinical placement.
- be competent at essential nursing skills.
- have time-management skills.
- take advantage of learning opportunities.
- be open to the suggestions and guidance offered.
- be aware of and practise within their scope of practice.
- have good interpersonal skills.
- practise according to occupational health and safety (OH&S) guidelines.
- understand the importance of accurate documentation and other legal and ethical issues.
- come to the clinical placement adequately prepared (with clear and realistic clinical learning objectives).

Do these expectations seem realistic to you or a pretty tall order? How do you measure up? It is always interesting, and sometimes surprising, to see a situation from another person's perspective. When the situation is as important as your clinical placement experience, it is vital that you consider it from many perspectives. We've spent time with many students who were really not aware of what clinicians expected of them and were puzzled and often hurt by the feedback they received.

We have not listed any coaching tips in this section—there are plenty of strategies scattered through this book that will provide the guidance and ideas to meet these expectations.

Tips and tales 2.3
Professional expectations

In Australia the professional expectations of nurses are spelt out very clearly. Nurses are required to provide high-quality care through safe and effective clinical practice. National standards of nursing practice have been developed by the Australian Nursing and Midwifery Council (ANMC). These standards are reviewed regularly to ensure that they are reflective of contemporary practice. The standards include:

- The National Competency Standards for the Registered Nurse
- The Code of Ethics for Nurses in Australia
- The Code of Professional Conduct for Nurses in Australia

These standards communicate to the general public, particularly healthcare consumers, the knowledge, skills, behaviours, attitudes and values expected of nurses. These are the professional expectations that form the framework against which your practice will be assessed. You will be required to demonstrate that you have met these standards as an indication that you are fit to provide safe, competent care in a variety of· settings. Your ability to meet these standards determines your eligibility for registration.

Each state and territory has regulatory authorities that maintain standards and processes for initial and ongoing registration. These are the organisations to which you will apply for registration once you have completed your course. You cannot practise as a registered nurse unless you are registered.

The ANMC National Competency Standards for the Registered Nurse (2005)

The National Competency Standards for the Registered Nurse have established a national benchmark for registered nurses and reinforce responsibility and accountability in delivering quality nursing care through safe and effective work practice.

The competencies that make up the ANMC National Competency Standards for the Registered Nurse are organised into four domains:

1. Professional practice

This relates to the professional, legal and ethical responsibilities that require demonstration of a satisfactory knowledge base, accountability for practice, functioning in accordance with legislation affecting nursing and healthcare, and the protection of individual and group rights.

2. Critical thinking and analysis

This relates to self-appraisal, professional development, and the value of evidence and research for practice. Reflecting on practice, feelings and beliefs and the consequences of these for individuals or groups is an important professional benchmark.

3. Provision and coordination of care

This domain relates to the coordination, organisation and provision of nursing care that includes the assessment of individuals or groups, planning, implementation and evaluation of care.

4. Collaborative and therapeutic practice

This relates to establishing, sustaining and concluding professional relationships with individuals or groups. This also contains those competencies that relate to nurses' understanding of their contribution to interdisciplinary healthcare.

Code of Ethics for Nurses in Australia (2002)

The Code of Ethics outlines the nursing profession's intention to accept the rights of individuals and to uphold these rights in practice. The Code of Ethics is complementary to the International Council of Nurses (ICN) Code of Ethics for Nurses (2000).

Purpose

* To identify the fundamental moral commitments of the profession.
* To provide nurses with a basis for reflection on ethical conduct, both as a professional and as an individual.
* To act as a guide to ethical practice.
* To indicate to the community the moral values that nurses can be expected to hold.

Value statements that comprise the Code of Ethics

* Nurses respect individual's needs, values, culture and vulnerability in the provision of nursing care.
* Nurses accept the rights of individuals to make informed choices in relation to their care.
* Nurses promote and uphold the provision of quality nursing care for all people.
* Nurses hold in confidence any information obtained in a professional capacity, use professional judgment where there is a need to share information for the therapeutic benefit and safety of a person, and ensure that privacy is safeguarded.
* Nurses fulfil the accountability and responsibility inherent in their roles.

The Code of Professional Conduct for Nurses in Australia (2003)

The Code of Professional Conduct for Nurses in Australia is a set of expected national standards of nursing conduct for Australian nurses. The code is not intended to give detailed professional advice on specific issues and areas of practice; rather, it identifies the minimum requirements for conduct in the profession. A breach of the code may constitute professional misconduct or unprofessional conduct.

The nursing profession expects that nurses will conduct themselves personally and professionally in a way that will maintain public trust and confidence in the profession. Nurses have a responsibility to the individual, society and the profession to provide safe and competent nursing care that is responsive to individual, group and community needs, and to the profession. A nurse must:

- practise in a safe and competent manner.
- practise in accordance with the agreed standards of the profession.
- not bring discredit upon the reputation of the nursing profession.
- practise in accordance with laws relevant to the nurse's area of practice.
- respect the dignity, culture, values and beliefs of an individual and any significant other person.
- support the health, wellbeing and informed decision-making of an individual.
- promote and preserve the trust that is inherent in the privileged relationship between a nurse and an individual, and respect both the person and property of that individual.
- treat personal information obtained in a professional capacity as confidential.
- refrain from engaging in exploitation, misinformation and misrepresentation in regard to healthcare products and nursing services.

It is essential that you become very familiar with each of the ANMC National standards. We have provided only the briefest overview of these standards here. The full documents (The National Competency Standard for Registered and Enrolled Nurses, The Code of Ethics for Nurses in Australia and The Code of Professional Conduct for Nurses in Australia) are available from the ANMC website: <http://www.anmc.org.au>.

Tips and tales 2.4
Don't apologise for being a student

There are three aspects that we'd like to focus on in this section—being proud to be a nurse (or a nursing student), behaving in a way that demonstrates that pride, and apologising for being a student. So many times students respond to questions from clients, doctors and nursing staff with a self-deprecating answer. When asked: 'What do you do?', 'Who are you?' or 'What is your position?' a student often answers, 'Oh, I'm *just a student*'. Likewise, we've heard students (and registered nurses) say to patients, 'Hello. I'm Jill and I'll be looking after you today'. Nurses do so much more than simply *look after* clients. The nursing profession is a proud profession (and rightly so), but for too long nurses have failed to demonstrate real pride in who they are and what they do.

You may not be a registered nurse (yet), or an employee of the institution, but you do have a right to be there, to engage in client-centred activities, to ask questions and to learn. You do not need to apologise for being a student or for being in the clinical learning environment. In fact you should be proud of your role and the valuable contribution that you make.

Coaching tips

- Practise sharing with others who you are and what you do, in a succinct and professional manner. Put a positive spin on your statements and express pride in your role as a student nurse: for example, 'I am Jill Jones. I'm a third-year nursing student from the University of —. I'll be working with Bill Smith today and we'll be responsible for your care'.
- Don't apologise when you cannot undertake a clinical skill or activity that you have not previously learnt. Simply explain that you have not been taught that particular skill, but that you would value the opportunity to watch the registered nurse undertake the procedure.
- Similarly, don't apologise when you are asked to do something that you are not legally permitted to do: for example, titrating intravenous fluids without supervision. Explain your program requirements and scope of practice, and politely decline to undertake the procedure.
- Don't apologise for asking questions or for the extra time that mentoring a student takes. Certainly acknowledge and appreciate this, but be mindful that in many respects students are an asset to the clinical staff they work with.
- Lastly, give the people you work with and the clients you are responsible for the respect they deserve, and expect to be treated with respect in return.

Tips and tales 2.5
Speak up, speak out

Standing up for what you believe in is one of the most important aspects of personal integrity. Yet speaking up or speaking out is not always easy. Traditionally nursing students were socialised to obedience, respect for authority and loyalty to the team. Their acceptance into, and continued membership of, the healthcare

Something to think about...

To everything there is a season, and a time to every purpose under heaven: a time to keep silence, and a time to speak.
Ecclesiastes 3:1

team depended upon their recognition of this subordinate role (Kelly 1996). Nearly a century ago Florence Nightingale described the qualities of a 'good nurse' as 'restraint, discipline and obedience. She [the nurse] should carry out the orders of the doctors in a suitably humble and deferential way. She should obey to the letter the requirements of the matron and the sister' (Davies 1977). Society expected nurses to be servile, subordinate, humble and self-sacrificing. Within the hierarchy of the healthcare system, nurses became acculturated to do and say what was expected, to conform rather than to question, to accept rather than debate important issues.

Nurses are shaking off this outdated image of nursing, and there are glimpses of a new era on the horizon. But for some it is a slow and difficult journey. Little wonder, then, that even today some nursing students find it difficult to speak out when their acceptance into the team may hinge on their conformity to it. There is nothing wrong with wanting to fit in and be accepted—it is a natural social phenomenon (Baumeister & Leary 1995). However, when fitting in becomes more important than doing what is right, it can become an ethical dilemma. The greatest threat to personal integrity is silence in the face of perceived wrong. We sometimes fail to consider the price of silence. To know something is wrong and to say nothing indirectly consents to what has occurred. In doing nothing we become part of the problem. This presents an enormous dilemma for students. By speaking out you may risk ridicule, rejection or social isolation. By not speaking out you may compromise your integrity.

Coaching tips

Many situations may present ethical dilemmas for student nurses. Horizontal violence (or bullying), compromised clinical practice or breaches of legal and/or ethical standards may call upon you to take a stand and to speak out. How will you respond? What will you say?

The ability to state your opinion clearly and honestly without offending anyone requires great skill. Start by using 'I' statements. Griffin (2004) provides some excellent examples of 'I' statements for when horizontal violence looms its ugly head:

- 'I don't feel right talking about him/her when I wasn't there and I don't know all the facts.'
- 'I'm not prepared to talk about it as it was shared in confidence.'
- 'I don't think that was what really happened—let's ask the people involved.'

Concerns about patient care standards are just as challenging and often need to be interpreted in consultation with an experienced and objective support person, such as your clinical educator. Be careful! Sometimes what may seem at first to be poor practice may not be so when interpreted in the light of all the facts. Don't jump in without some guidance and knowledge of all the pertinent issues. You can still use 'I' statements, but be tactful in your approach. 'I don't understand the reason for that decision' is often a wise opening statement that allows for lines of communication to remain open and for explanations to be provided.

There may come a time when you feel you must speak out strongly against a clinical, ethical or professional issue. Make sure you are familiar with and guided by the Code of Ethics (ANMC 2002), which provides guidelines for nurses. As a student you may need to call upon your support networks, clinical educators or educational institution staff for guidance and advice. In some situations they may need to advocate on your behalf.

Speaking up or speaking out is an act of moral courage. It often carries a price tag. But an even greater price tag comes with silence— the loss of self-respect. The benefits of speaking up outweigh the risks, not only from a personal point of view but also for the nursing profession (Kelly 1996).

When in doubt about whether you should speak out, reflect on the words of Martin Luther King Junior: 'He who passively accepts evil is as much involved in it as he who helps to perpetrate it. He who accepts evil without protesting against it is really cooperating with it.'

Tips and tales 2.6
Exercise your rights

On campus, clinical placements and even in this book, you'll hear a great deal about your responsibilities. Always keep in mind that alongside responsibilities there are also rights. Nurses have focused on their responsibilities for so long that they are often surprised at the prospect of having rights themselves. Rights always seem to belong to other people—human rights, patient rights, women's rights, consumer rights—the list goes on. It's time to think about your rights as a nursing student. In this section we'll touch on a few of your rights and provide some strategies to help you to exercise these rights.

Coaching tips

1. The right to ask questions

As a student your primary purpose in undertaking a clinical placement is to learn. This won't happen unless you ask questions. Some of the nurses you work with will welcome your questions. These nurses should be congratulated for supporting your learning. Unfortunately, some nurses imply that students ask too many questions.

It's your right to ask questions, but always ask at the right time and in the right place. To develop your problem-solving skills, attempt to work through the question first and develop a tentative answer yourself. For example, you could ask your mentor if your patient's urine output needs to be measured. Alternatively you could check the patient's chart, look for a fluid balance chart, reflect on what may have been said at handover (did you take notes?) and consider the patient's diagnosis (renal failure, congestive cardiac failure etc). Doing this allows you to demonstrate initiative and develop an 'informed' question. For example, 'I've measured Mrs Smith's urine output and tested the specific gravity because she has renal failure. Would you like me to document the amount on her fluid balance chart?'

2. The right to question practice

This is a right that nursing students don't always exercise. You will learn about 'best practice' and 'evidence-based practice' (and we discuss it in Chapter 3), but at times you will see nursing practice that seems to be based on little more than authority ('The doctor said to do it this way'), tradition ('We've always done it this way') and local policy ('This is the way we do it here'). You may find yourself placed in a confusing and somewhat uncomfortable position with this contradiction between theory and practice.

On completing a central line dressing, one student asked, 'Why is this central line being dressed daily with a gauze dressing? Everything I've read suggests that a transparent dressing that stays on for up to 7 days is the ideal dressing product for central lines'. Now if you've done any reading about central lines, you'll know that this student was absolutely right! Her comment promoted a lot of dialogue and debate among the registered nurses and doctors. Not too much later, following a review of the literature, the central-line dressing regime was updated at that hospital. You guessed it—transparent dressings are now used. When questioning practice, be tactful and polite; there may be very sound reasons for the way nursing procedures are undertaken.

3. The right of refusal (without feeling guilty or making excuses)

Often when students refuse a request from a superior they feel guilty and uncomfortable, even when they are within their rights, and even when it is their responsibility to refuse. Here is an example in which a nurse refused, politely and tactfully, but with determination:

Registered nurse: You can go and administer the oral medications to the patient in room 11. I trust you.

Student: Thank you for trusting me to do this on my own, but as a student I'm required to have the administration of all medications counter-checked, witnessed and countersigned by the nurse responsible for the patient's care. I can fail my clinical placement if I don't comply with this policy.

---

4. The right to be supernumerary to the workforce

Since nursing education moved to institutions of higher education, students have undertaken clinical placements in a supernumerary capacity. This means that you are not part of the workforce but are there *in addition* to the employed staff. This is so that your learning is not compromised by the demands and responsibilities of patient care. However, occasionally students, particularly when in third year, are used to fill a gap in the roster. While we encourage students to take a patient load, it should always be under the supervision of the nurse responsible for the patient's care. If this situation presents itself, politely explain your educational institution's policy.

Tips and tales 2.7
You're not the boss of me (oh really?)

As you step into your next ward, excited and ready to begin your clinical placement, the nursing unit manager (NUM) will be there, standing at the door, smiling in welcome, eager for you to feel wanted and needed. The NUM will spend much time complimenting you on your skills and making wonderful comments about you to the other staff. She or he will most definitely understand if you are late for your shift because of car problems, or not in correct uniform because you 'forgot' to do the washing, or if you seem a little tired or unmotivated; after all nursing is a difficult and tiring occupation and special allowances do need to be made for students. Reality check! Nursing unit managers are busy people. Their first responsibility is patient welfare. NUMs are responsible for budgets, equipment, resources, standards of practice, occupational health and safety, rostering, staffing issues and problems, quality management, infection control—the list goes on. Students are one of the many important considerations for NUMs. They will expect you to meet the same professional standards as their staff in terms of presentation, punctuality, work ethics, standards of practice etc.

We've heard students complain when they have been reminded by the NUM 'not to be late', to 'wear the correct uniform', or to 'tie their hair up'. Some students believe that because they are not employees the NUM has no authority over them. You need to be aware that you are a guest in each clinical venue. The NUM is responsible for all that occurs in the unit, is committed to maintaining high professional practice standards and has the final say on who does (and does not) undertake a placement there.

Coaching tips

There are many different leadership styles. No two NUMS are alike. Some are hands-on, delving into patient care whenever they get the chance. Others prefer to delegate. Some are social, warm and chatty; others are quiet and distant. However, there are some consistencies that you should be aware of:

- Most managers don't like surprises and don't like to be told about the deterioration of a patient's condition after it has already happened. They want to know if a difficult situation is developing with a patient, rather than have to face an emergency as they are about to go home. NUMs like to be kept informed. Whether equipment is faulty, a patient's false teeth are missing or the cleaners have gone on strike, the 'buck stops' with the NUM and he or she needs to be kept informed.
- Most NUMs don't like to be presented with a problem, complaint or concern without some form of proposed solution. It is important to remember that they try to be fair, but they are accountable to the patients, staff, doctors and the administration. Sometimes they really are the 'meat in the sandwich', as there are so many people they must try to satisfy. Managers need to take a global perspective, so be understanding when your needs are not their first priority.
- Many NUMS prefer the direct approach. Nothing is more disconcerting (and likely to cause tension and distrust) than hearing about problems through rumours, innuendo and gossip. The direct approach allows for face-to-face discussion of feelings and issues. Choose the most appropriate time and place to bring up difficult or controversial issues.
- Assertiveness is a good communication skill; however, ensure that your information is correct before you speak (and avoid aggressive outbursts).

Tips and tales 2.8
Don't take everything personally

The clinical learning environment is a complex social setting (Hughes 2002) and presents countless challenges to students. Some of these you will find exhilarating and others will provide you with experiences that will improve your interpersonal skills. Accepting constructive feedback from staff and educators about your behaviour during challenging situations will add to your growth and development. Avoid taking things personally. Some situations nurses find themselves in are not always planned, and it is helpful to consider each situation as a clinical issue or problem, rather than something that is a personal attack or problem for you.

Remember that all situations create learning, and through learning we change and grow, develop new skill sets, knowledge and attitudes, and re-evaluate our belief systems. Identify what it is you know and what it is that you need to seek help with. Compare each situation with previous learning situations and your observations of experienced staff.

Consider this example by a student who demonstrated less than appropriate professional behaviour, following a directive from her clinical educator.

Evelyn wanted to go to theatre, but she was told by her clinical educator that she was to remain on the medical ward because the perioperative unit already had a group of students. During lunch break, Evelyn found out that another student in her group had been to theatre that morning with her patient. She went to her clinical educator complaining that she had stopped her from achieving one of her goals and that she was favouring other students. Discussions about the situation between Evelyn and her clinical educator became strained when Evelyn could not understand why she couldn't go to the unit when her colleague had done so. Evelyn saw

*the issue as one that was a personal attack on her and
complained to university staff about the way she was treated
by the clinical educator.*

*On examination of the issues surrounding the complaint,
the university staff identified that eight students from another
university were allocated to the perioperative environment. Students
from the ward locations were permitted to visit the perioperative
environment only if they accompanied the patients they were caring
for. As Evelyn was on a medical ward, none of her patients were
scheduled for theatre.*

The very nature of the clinical environment is dynamic and
each student's learning experience will be different. It is not
beneficial to compare your experiences and opportunities to
those of other students, as no two experiences will ever be the
same. In the above situation, Evelyn's placement did not give
her the opportunity to go to the perioperative unit and it was
a professional decision taken by the educator, not a personal
attack .

Coaching tips

- Identify challenging or difficult situations and work through
  them using conflict resolution skills (see section 3.4).
- Seek out strategies to help you deal with difficult people or with
  difficult situations (counselling courses can be beneficial to help
  with the development of strategies).
- Be aware of your own behaviours, how you react to situations
  and how you work through issues.
- Seek assistance from mentors, educators and other relevant staff,
  as necessary, to work through situations in the clinical learning
  environment.

Tips and tales 2.9
Compliance and compromise

This tale revisits the importance of belonging, but delves into the 'dark side' of this phenomenon for nursing students. There is a broad range of psychological literature that describes the importance of belonging, as well as the negative emotional, psychological, physical and behavioural consequences of having this need thwarted. The absence of meaningful interpersonal work relationships can lead to unquestioning agreement with other people's decisions, acquiescence, compliance or going along with negative behaviours sanctioned by group members in order to belong (Champion et al 1998; Clark 1992; Hart & Rotem 1994; Hemmings 1993).

What does this mean for nursing students? Some studies claim that for many students, the need to belong and to be accepted into the team is more important than the quality of care they provide and the level of competency they aspire to (Bradby 1990; Champion et al 1998; Tradewell 1996). *Reread that sentence a couple of times and ask yourself if it could apply to you.* Nursing students have described how they sometimes go along with clinical practices that they know to be wrong so as not to 'rock the boat'. They share how it is easier to just accept that 'this is the way it is done here' rather than be labelled a 'troublemaker.' Compare these notions with what you've learnt about questioning practices that are not evidence-based.

Coaching tips

We would like to give you a tried-and-tested recipe for overcoming the need to conform in order to belong, but really there is no simple solution. The best advice that we can offer is that you reflect on this section thoughtfully. At some stage you may be in a situation where you'll feel pressured to compromise your practice: think carefully about the consequences, for you and for your patient.

Something to think about...

Will you be a change agent or a conformist? Will you stand up for what you know to be right or will you bow to peer pressure?

Tips and tales 2.10
Being naive

Student nurses may not have cornered the market on naivety, but they often take what people say at face value. Some people find naivety refreshing in a person just beginning their career. It may motivate them to take the newcomer 'under their wing' and tell them 'how things work around here'. Students tend not to probe deeply to determine the veracity of what they're told, perhaps because they want to see the best in people, or because they don't feel it is their place to do so. Understandably, it is difficult to see the big picture when you are only on a placement for a short period of time.

Coaching tips

* Don't be 'too grateful' when the person who offers to 'show you the ropes', shares titbits of information that undermine other staff on the nursing team.
* Don't feel that you have to take sides or show allegiance to the person that 'takes you under their wing'. In fact, you should avoid this at all costs and maintain a neutral stance.
* Without assuming the worst, get into the habit of asking yourself what a person's motives might be.
* Don't rely on the word of just one person—always look at the 'big picture'. Gather as much information as possible.

- Trust your instincts—if you feel uncomfortable about what you're being told, it may be for good reason.
- Keep in mind that the type of person who undermines, criticises and gossips about other staff on the ward, may treat you the same way the next time your back is turned.

Reflective thinking activities

What is the most important piece of advice that you would give to students about to undertake their first clinical placement?

_____

_____

_____

_____

List your 10 tips for success when on a clinical placement:

1._____

_____

_____

2._____

_____

_____

3._____

_____

_____

4._____

_____

_____

5. _____

_____

_____

6. _____

_____

_____

7. _____

_____

_____

8. _____

_____

_____

9. _____

_____

_____

10. _____

_____

_____

Have you ever been in a clinical situation where you believed patient safety or quality care was compromised? What did you do? In hindsight would you (could you) have done anything differently?

_____

_____

_____

_____

References

ANMC 2002. Code of Ethics for Nurses in Australia, Australian Nursing and Midwifery Council. Online. Available <www.anmc.org.au>, 1 April 2006.

Baumeister R & Leary M 1995 The need to belong: desire for interpersonal attachments as a fundamental human motivation. Psychological Bulletin 117(3):497–529.

Bradby B 1990 Status passage into nursing: another view of the process of socialisation into nursing. Journal of Advanced Nursing 15:1220–1225.

Champion B, Ambler N & Keating D 1998 Fitting in: becoming an insider: a nursing perspective (unpublished report). Nurses Registration Board of New South Wales, Newcastle.

Clark C 1992 Deviant adolescent subcultures: assessment strategies and clinical interventions. Adolescence 27(106):283–293.

Davies C 1977 Continuities in the development of hospital nursing in Britain. Journal of Advanced Nursing 2(5):479–493.

Griffin M 2004 Teaching cognitive rehearsal as a shield for lateral violence: an intervention for newly licensed nurses. Journal of Continuing Education in Nursing 35(6):257–264.

Hart G & Rotem A 1994 The best and the worst: students' experiences of clinical education. Australian Journal of Advanced Nursing 11(3):26–33.

Hemmings L 1993 From student to nurse. Paper presented at the Research in Nursing: Turning Points conference. Proceedings of the National Conference, Glenelg.

Hughes C 2002 Issues in supervisory facilitation. Studies in Continuing Education 24(1):57–71.

Kelly B 1996 Speaking up: a moral obligation. Nursing Forum 31(2):31–34.

McCormack B, Manley K, Kitson A et al 1999 Towards practice development—vision or reality? Journal of Nursing Management 7:255–264.

Tradewell G 1996 Rites of passage: adaptation of nursing graduates to a hospital setting. Journal of Nursing Staff Development 12(4):183–189.

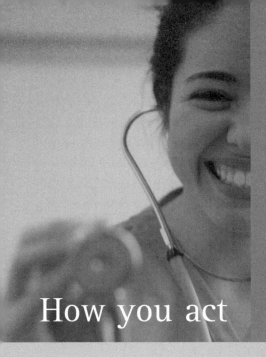

Chapter 3

How you act

Actions speak louder than words.

Proverb

Tips and tales 3.1
Cultural competence

An increase in cultural diversity in Australia has created the need for nurses to provide culturally competent care. This presents challenges for nurses to manage complex differences in communication, attitudes, religion, world views, theories and language (Kikuchi 2005; Schim et al 2005). The nurse theorist Madeleine Leininger (1991, p 36) defined culture as people's 'learned and transmitted values, beliefs and practices'. Cultural competence is described as 'the demonstration of knowledge, attitudes, and behaviours based on diverse, relevant, cultural experiences' (Schim et al 2005, p 355). Knowledge of others, therefore, is vitally important. To be culturally sensitive you need to recognise the attitudes, values, beliefs and practices within your own culture so that you can have an insight into your effect on others.

When you undertake clinical placements, cultural safety is essential to quality care. Culturally safe behaviour means making decisions based on principles such as justice and accountability. It centres on the experiences of the patient and is nested with an acceptance of human diversity (Kikuchi 2005; Schim et al 2005). In contrast, cultural competence depends on the capacity of the nurse to improve health by integrating culture into the clinical context.

Nursing students themselves represent a culturally diverse group. In different educational institutions, student populations reflect the social demographics. As a population, nursing students at any one Australian institution can be very culturally diverse. This provides you with the opportunity to gain knowledge and understanding of others and to integrate this into your nursing care. Despite many Australians living hybrid lives involving influences from many cultures, there is still a lot to learn from one another (Ang et al 2002). Consider this story.

Mrs Mana was a Maori woman who had been diagnosed with lung cancer. She had been admitted to hospital for palliative care. Within a few days the cancerous lesions had grown. She began to experience difficulty in breathing and underwent a procedure to remove fluid from her lung. She found the pleurocentesis (fluid tap procedure) very painful. Her doctor explained that the cancer was extremely fast-growing, and she was offered radiotherapy and chemotherapy. She was advised that these approaches would give her a little more time, but would not save her life.

Mrs Mana considered the treatment options and their associated side effects and discussed the issues with her daughters. Her main concern was the loss of hair that would result from the chemotherapy. Her cultural traditions included the belief that she must die as a whole person. She believed that without her hair she could not be considered to be a whole person. Together with her family's blessing, she declined the treatment that may have afforded her a longer life, so that she could die according to her cultural traditions.

What are your thoughts about Mrs Mana's decisions and her need to be true to her cultural beliefs?

Coaching tips

- Make cultural competence an everyday component of your practice. Incorporate cultural diversity (knowledge about the diversity in your healthcare area), awareness (knowledge of culture) and sensitivity (attitudes towards others) into your practice.
- Develop culturally competent behaviours by exposure to people from different cultures. Learn from others as you care for them.
- Examine policies and implement practices to promote culturally competent care.

- Promote cultural awareness and team building through open and respectful dialogue.
- Tailor your care to meet patients' social, cultural, religious and linguistic needs.
- Use interpreters for care requirements when language barriers are problematic (consider the sensitivity of the information that is being imparted by a third person).
- Respect personal space and conversational distance by using the appropriate tone of voice.
- Be attuned to non-verbal communication (body language), silence and touch.
- Use communication skills that reflect your sensitivity and willingness to listen to others.
- Accept and value difference and diversity in human behaviour, social structure and culture.

Tips and tales 3.2
The value of a smile

History proves the value of a smile. Studies indicate smiles are the oldest form of expressing the desire and willingness to cooperate. Smiles are potent facial expressions that can be detected from as far away as the far end of a football field, making them the most visible facial expressions from a distance.

The first thing that people usually notice when they meet someone for the first time is that person's smile. In fact, the majority of adults consider a person's smile to be very important at an initial meeting. Three out of four people think a smile is important for succeeding in the workplace. Considerer this scenario.

Not so long ago a group of clinicians were completing a student's clinical appraisal. The appraisal was very good and the student was considered competent, organised and knowledgable. He was punctual,

well presented, articulate, asked appropriate questions and worked hard.
However, the student's mentor commented, and the other staff agreed,
that she did not get the impression that the student had enjoyed the
clinical placement. He rarely smiled and a few patients had remarked
that he did not seem enthusiastic about being a nurse. When this
feedback was shared with him, he was taken by complete surprise.
He felt that this placement had been the best he'd had so far and he was
unaware that he had been perceived in this way. He admitted he was very
serious about being a good nurse, but did not realise that his seriousness
would be interpreted by others as a lack of enthusiasm and enjoyment.

Coaching tips

When we are in a new environment we often wait until someone
smiles at us before we offer a smile. Don't wait—a smile encourages
others to communicate with us. It can reassure and show empathy
to an anxious relative, comfort a distressed child, show support
and encouragement to an apprehensive or weary colleague, and
welcome a newcomer.

You might be enjoying your clinical placement, but fail to show
it. Your face should express what you feel when you wish to connect
with others. We are not encouraging you to smile inappropriately or
without spontaneity. Just be mindful of how important smiling is,
how it can break down barriers and how others will interpret your
smile as a sign of enthusiasm.

Tips and tales 3.3
Teamwork

Introducing the concept of 'teamwork' is difficult without resorting
to platitudes and rhetoric. No doubt as a student nurse you have
heard a lot about teams and the importance of teamwork. You
have probably worked hard to make sure that you fit into the

team. Before long you will graduate and be called upon to be a team leader. But what does teamwork really mean and what is the secret to successful teams? Life lessons are often found in nature. The story of geese (author unknown) is a tale that will provide enlightenment to this sometimes nebulous concept that we call teamwork.

Tale 1

As each goose flaps its wings it creates 'uplift' for the birds that follow. By flying in a 'V' formation, the whole flock achieves a greater flying range than if each bird flew alone.

Coaching tips

There is a lot that we can achieve on our own, even more can be achieved with the help of colleagues, but the power of what can be achieved by a team is quantum. People who share a common direction achieve great things because they are travelling on the trust of one another. The real world of the nurse is challenging and sometimes difficult. Effective teamwork is essential to nursing because it is the support mechanism that 'lifts and carries' us when we struggle. Alone the problems seem insurmountable; together anything is achievable.

Tale 2

When a goose falls out of formation, it suddenly feels the drag and resistance of flying alone. It quickly moves back into formation to take advantage of the lifting power of the bird immediately in front.

Coaching tips

If we had as much sense as geese we'd be willing to stay in formation with those who are headed in our direction, be willing to accept their help and advice and to give our support to others. It is difficult being a 'one man show' and there is strength in numbers. Giving help to and receiving help from fellow students and nursing colleagues is what makes a team and makes the impossible seem possible.

Tale 3

When the lead goose tires, it rotates back into formation and another goose flies to the point position.

Coaching tips

Don't be afraid to take the lead and to encourage others. Your leadership may be specific to patient care or provide motivation and a positive direction for the group.

Tale 4

The geese flying in formation honk to encourage those up front to keep up their speed.

Coaching tips

Let others know that they are doing a good job or that you appreciate their feedback. Be positive and encouraging.

Tale 5

When a goose gets sick, wounded or shot down, two geese drop out of formation and follow it down to help protect and care for it. They stay with it until it dies or is able to fly again. Then, they launch out with another formation or catch up with the flock.

Coaching tips

The art of caring is a wondrous human trait. Reach out to others, and show empathy and support to colleagues and peers.

Tips and tales 3.4
Managing conflict

Conflict is inevitable and occurs in every workplace and in any relationship. Conflict is difficult and distressing, but it does provide the opportunity for stimulating discussion and for developing your interpersonal skills. Sometimes conflict arises because of a misuse of power, authoritarian tactics or condescension, sometimes it is the result of a misunderstanding or miscommunication, while at other times it is simply a personality clash.

Coaching tips

- Ask yourself if you have done anything to contribute to the conflict. Try to be objective and to look at the problem from all sides.
- Keep things in perspective. This will usually require you to spend some time alone to put your thoughts in order. If the issue is not worth losing sleep over, let it go.
- Confer with the other person in a neutral and private setting (not in the nurses' station).
- Share your thoughts and feelings. Explain the problem from your perspective: 'I feel…', or 'It seems to me…'.
- Check your understanding. Listen to the other person's perspective. Try to understand the reasons behind the conflict.
- Look for common ground and attempt a compromise. Pursue a good outcome for all involved. If the other person sees that you are willing to make some changes to achieve reconciliation, they will hopefully meet you half way.
- Try not to become defensive or use personal attacks.
- Use direct confrontation as a last resort.
- Talk to other students about similar experiences and how they handled them.

- Decide upon a course of action. If a satisfactory compromise cannot be reached, you'll need to make a difficult choice. If you decide to yield to another person's decision, do so without self-pity and resentment. If you decide to stand up for your rights, be aware of relevant policies, the appropriate steps to take, and who to speak to (for example, mentors, clinical educators, lecturers, or counsellors).

Other considerations

Sometimes other factors affect how you view the situation. Consider whether you are:

- fatigued—have you been taking care of yourself properly? Could your tiredness be making you unreasonable?
- stressed—is there something happening in your personal life that is overshadowing your ability to see the situation clearly?

Tips and tales 3.5
Dealing with horizontal violence

Although many nurses may not be familiar with the term horizontal violence, most have experienced it (and participated in it) at some time during their career. The concept of horizontal violence or bullying has been discussed in the nursing literature for almost two decades. It is defined as nurses covertly or overtly directing their dissatisfaction towards each other and to those less powerful than themselves (Griffin 2004). It has been suggested that because nurses are dominated (and, by implication, oppressed) by a patriarchal system headed by doctors, administrators and nurse managers, nurses lower down the hierarchy of power resort to aggression among themselves (Farrell 1997, p 482). There are many obvious manifestations of horizontal violence, and others that are quite subtle.

The 10 most frequent forms of horizontal violence in nursing (adapted from Duffy 1995 and Farrell 1997) are the following:

- non-verbal innuendo (raising of eyebrows, pulling faces)
- verbal affront (snide remarks, abrupt responses)
- undermining activities (turning away, not being available, exclusion)
- withholding information (about practice or patients)
- sabotage (deliberately setting up a negative situation)
- infighting (bickering with peers)
- scapegoating (attributing all that goes wrong to one individual)
- backstabbing (complaining to others about an individual instead of speaking directly to that individual)
- failure to respect privacy
- broken confidences

Horizontal violence is one of the most personally troubling experiences for nurses. Internationally it is claimed that one in three nurses leave their position because of workplace bullying (Griffin 2004). Students undertaking a clinical placement have been identified as a group that is especially vulnerable to horizontal violence. One reason for this vulnerability is their inexperience, which makes their work subject to scrutiny and criticism. Horizontal violence can cause students significant stress, and prevent them from asking questions and feeling as if they fit in. Sometimes registered nurses excuse their behaviour by saying, 'This is how people treated me when I was a student'.

Coaching tips

Understanding the origins and extent of horizontal violence in nursing will help you realise that you are not to blame and that you should not take it personally. It is also important that you learn how to break the cycle of horizontal violence by confronting the situation rather than trying to ignore it. Confrontation is difficult but often results in the resolution of the bullying behaviour.

How to confront horizontal violence

Here are some examples of how to confront horizontal violence (adapted from Griffin 2004):

Action: Non-verbal innuendo *(raised eyebrows, face pulling)*
Response: 'I sense from your facial expression that there may be something you wish to say to me. It is fine to speak to me directly.'

Action: Verbal affront *(snide remarks or abrupt response)*
Response: 'I learn best from people who can give me clear and complete directions and feedback. Could I ask you to be more open with me?'

Action: Backstabbing
Response: 'I don't feel comfortable talking behind his/her back.' *(Then walk away.)*

Action: Broken confidences
Response: 'I thought that was shared in confidence.'

Appropriate behaviours

Here are some appropriate behaviours for those who consider themselves to be professional (adapted from Chaska 2000):

- Respect the privacy of others.
- Be willing to help when asked.
- Keep confidences.
- Work cooperatively despite feelings of dislike.
- Don't undermine or criticise colleagues.

- Address colleagues by name, and ask for help and advice when needed.
- Look colleagues in the eye when having a conversation.
- Don't be overly inquisitive about other people's lives.
- Don't engage in conversation about a colleague with another colleague.
- Stand up for a colleague in a conversation if he or she is not present.
- Don't exclude people from conversations or social activities.
- Don't criticise publicly.

Tips and tales 3.6
Dealing with sexual harassment

Some authorities contend that the nursing profession has the highest rate of sexual harassment (Madison & Minichicello 2001). Sexual harassment is perpetuated by both staff and patients and comes in many guises. Many people tolerate it, some hardly notice it, and some find it amusing in small doses and even laugh about it.

Stereotypical images of nurses have played a contributing part in sexual harassment. Media images of nurses are improving but in the past nurses were often stereotyped as being flirtatious and sometimes sexually promiscuous. Male nurses have been stereotyped too. They are sometimes victimised for doing what for years was considered to be 'women's work'.

What one person interprets as sexual harassment can be considered by another as a 'bit of harmless fun'. Harassment can run the gamut from offensive jokes or sexual comments to inappropriate touching. Sexual assaults are rare but do occur. The overwhelming majority of sexual harassment cases are between male patients and female nurses (Hamlin & Hoffman 2002). Such harassment creates tension for nurses, who must walk a fine line between meeting their professional responsibilities to patients and protecting themselves.

What is sexual harassment?

Sexual harassment is characterised by conduct of a sexual nature that is unwanted and unwelcome to the receiver. Conduct is considered unwelcome when it is neither invited nor solicited, and the behaviour is deemed offensive and undesirable. Sexual harassment in the workplace is an unlawful exercise of power where the harasser uses his or her authority or power to belittle, intimidate or humiliate.

Based on Hamlin & Hoffman 2002

Harassing behaviours may include the following (Gardner & Johnson 2001):
- verbal sexual advances determined by the recipient as unwelcome
- sexually oriented comments about someone's body, appearance and/or lifestyle
- offensive behaviour, such as leering, ridicule or innuendo
- display of offensive visual materials
- deliberate unwanted physical contact

Coaching tips

As a nurse you should be vigilant against sexual harassment. If someone speaks or acts inappropriately towards you this is what you can do:

- Recognise the behaviour.
- Don't blame yourself.
- Keep a diary of what has happened.
- Tell the person involved that you are uncomfortable with this behaviour and that it offends or scares you. Some people do not realise the effect of their behaviour and are genuinely horrified when they are told that their actions are perceived to be harassing when they thought they were being friendly or amusing. Offenders need to understand that is it not what they intended that matters, but how they are perceived.

- Take yourself out of the situation. If a person seems to be targeting you inappropriately, ensure that you are never alone with them.
- Give no encouragement. If someone is harassing you, don't respond to them. Do not engage in friendly banter.
- Confide in a colleague if you think someone is harassing you, even if it is only minor pestering.
- Know the policies and procedures of the educational and healthcare institutions about harassment.
- If the situation escalates, report the offender to your educator, mentor or nursing unit manager who can take appropriate action.
- If a patient speaks to you or touches you inappropriately, challenge the person immediately in a firm, clear, loud voice for other people to hear. If the harassment continues, you can ask to have another nurse stand by in the patient's room, or refuse to care for the patient. Regardless of what you do, you should report the behaviour to a superior.

Remember that sexual harassment is against the law. All educational and healthcare institutions have policies to protect against sexual harassment. Do not tolerate it (or perpetuate it) in any form.

Tips and tales 3.7
Taking care of yourself

Nursing students are a healing presence to others. It is essential that you care for yourself to enable you to continue to care for others and to practise safe nursing (Stark et al 2005). Caring for yourself requires that you proactively adopt healthier lifestyle choices. Practising healthier lifestyle options will maintain and enhance your health and wellness and put you in the best possible position to cope with the demands of nursing. You are responsible for your own health, and a holistic assessment of your health and wellbeing will help you to identify your needs and any problems that require a change in lifestyle. Arm yourself with knowledge about health and wellness, select appropriate strategies and commit to making health choices.

Caring for yourself needs to be a priority before you can care for others. The major components of a healthy lifestyle are physical activity, nutrition, interpersonal relations, spiritual growth and stress management (Stark et al 2005). As a role model for others you should exemplify a healthy lifestyle.

Coaching tips

- Eat well. Get enough rest. Exercise regularly. Be kind to yourself. Take a few minutes each day just to reflect and dream in solitude. Take this time to renew yourself physically, mentally, emotionally, and spiritually. Private time is not a luxury—it is a necessity.
- Assess and analyse your own health. Set up a personalised plan that addresses your needs and problems. Seek professional health advice as necessary. Many gyms will assist you with health advice.
- Ensure that you are familiar with the immunisation require-ments of your state or territory's health department. Most uni-versities require you to have evidence of having complied with these requirements before you are authorised to begin your clinical placements.
- Manual handling injuries are one of the most common reasons for nurses' absenteeism. It is vitally important that you learn safe manual handling techniques and practise these at all times.
- You'll learn a lot about infection control during your studies. Remember that infection control protects both your patients and you!

- Remember that you are only human. This is your greatest strength and greatest weakness. Learn to say no to people who put excessive demands upon you. Learn to say yes to activities you really enjoy.
- Develop time-management skills to help you juggle study, friends, family and work. Prioritise and don't leave things to the last minute (the extra stress is just not worth it).
- Implement strategies to lessen the effects of lifestyle and work stressors. Try to eliminate as many of these stressors as possible (for example, learn progressive relaxation).
- Set up support networks with colleagues for clinical placement. These can include childcare support networks, travel groups and study groups. You will need to be proactive to work on this.
- Talk about your clinical experiences with each other (remember confidentiality and privacy requirements)—this is a great debriefing mechanism as well as an affirming strategy.
- Seek help and support early in your placement experience if you perceive a problem. It is better to deal with issues early than to allow them to escalate.

Tips and tales 3.8
Patient advocacy

Patient advocacy is an essential responsibility for all health professionals—it is no less an obligation for students. To be an advocate means that you should empower and uphold the rights and interests of others. Patient advocacy is defined as an ethical principle of beneficence and is 'defending the rights of the vulnerable patient, or acting on behalf of those unable to assert their rights' (Thompson et al 2000, p 20). Ways to advocate for and to empower others could include the following:

- informing a patient of her or his rights
- helping a patient to explore options

- helping patients to help themselves
- speaking on behalf of a patient (if and when requested)
- assisting patients to express their views clearly and confidently
- investigating and following up on complaints

As well as acting as advocate for others, you may require an advocate yourself at times during your nursing career. In some circumstances your clinical educator may be able to advocate on your behalf, or your lecturer may be the person who can best represent your interests. Do not hesitate to request this type of support. You should also be aware that there are professional advocates available, and a search of websites (for example, of professional groups, nurses' associations and colleges of nursing) will identify services available to nurses.

Coaching tips

- Identify the essential human rights that a nurse must respect in order to be a patient advocate.
- Identify your responsibilities as a patient advocate.
- Carefully gather relevant information related to the situation and patient before addressing an issue. Try to stand back from the personal and analyse all issues objectively.
- Use placement feedback mechanisms to provide information about facilities (that is, evaluations) on all occasions; feedback, whether good or bad, contributes to improved practices.
- Empower patients to self-advocate rather than taking over (that is, allow patients to ask their own questions of members of the interdisciplinary healthcare team). Perhaps set the scene so that patients are able to ask their questions or suggest they write their questions down before a consultation.
- Provide patients with information that enables them to make informed decisions.
- Speak up and seek support for your concerns from your clinical educator, mentor or academic staff.

- Discuss issues of concern with your mentor or nursing unit manager. If you feel uncomfortable, request a support person to be present during the meeting.
- Avoid the use of confrontational actions (such as speaking with media or others).
- Use the support of lecturers to work through issues and principles that you may be concerned about—follow educational institution policies and procedures related to clinical practicum.

Tips and tales 3.9
Best practice

Something to think about...

The true journey of discovery does not consist of searching for new territories, but in having new eyes.
Marcel Proust (French novelist, 1871–1922)

Often when we visit students on a clinical placement we ask them questions like 'What are you doing?' 'Why are you doing it?' 'Why are you doing it that way?' 'Is there a better way?' We're always thrilled if they can provide evidence-based justification for their decisions. So often nursing care is based upon little more than tradition or authority. Let us explain.

As a nursing student you will learn how to practise nursing, and some (hopefully most) of what you learn will be research-based. Millenson (1997) estimates, however, that 85 per cent of healthcare practice has not been scientifically validated. Nursing practice relies on a collage of information sources that vary in dependability and validity, and some sources of evidence and knowledge are more important than others (Dawes et al 2005). Let us consider some of these sources.

Sources of evidence and knowledge

Tradition

In the nursing profession certain beliefs are accepted as facts and certain practices are accepted as effective, based purely on custom and tradition. These traditions and customs may be so entrenched that their use and usefulness is not questioned or rigorously evaluated. It is worrying when 'unit culture' (the way it is done here) determines the way practice is undertaken, rather than basing clinical judgment on the best available evidence.

Authority

Another common source of knowledge is an authority figure, a person with specialised expertise and/or in a position of authority. Reliance on the advice of authority figures such as nursing managers, educators or academics is understandable. However, like tradition, these authorities as a source of information have limitations. Authorities are not infallible (especially if their knowledge is based mainly on personal experience), yet their knowledge often goes unchallenged.

Clinical experience

Clinical experience is a familiar and important source of knowledge. The ability to recognise regularities and irregularities, to generalise and to make predictions based on observations is a hallmark of good nursing practice. Nevertheless, personal experience has limitations also. Individual experiences and perspectives are sometimes narrow and biased.

Intuition

Nurses sometimes rely on 'intuition' in their practice. Intuition is a form of knowledge that cannot be explained on the basis of reasoning or prior instruction. Although intuition and 'hunches' undoubtedly play a role in nursing practice, it is inappropriate to depend solely on these feelings as a source of evidence for practice.

Trial and error

Sometimes we tackle problems by successively trying out alternative solutions. While this approach may in some cases be practical, it is often fallible and inefficient, to say nothing of the ethical implications of trial and error in clinical practice. This method tends to be haphazard, and the solutions are often idiosyncratic.

Assembled information

In making clinical decisions, healthcare professionals may use information that has been assembled for various purposes. For example, local, national and international benchmarking data provides information on the rates of various procedures and/or related complications (such as hospital-acquired infections). Risk-management data such as critical incident reports and medication error reports can be used to assess and measure improvements in practice. However, they do not always provide the actual knowledge needed to implement improvement.

Evidence-based research

Nurses are increasingly expected to adopt an evidence-based practice approach, which can be defined as the use of the *best* clinical evidence available to inform patient care decisions. Evidence from rigorous studies constitutes the best type of evidence for underpinning nurses' decisions, actions and interactions with patients. Nursing care that is based upon high-quality research evidence is more likely to be cost-effective and result in positive outcomes (Joanna Briggs Institute 2004).

The need for evidence to support practice has never been greater. The knowledge on which nursing care is based is constantly changing and some of what you are taught in your nursing program will rapidly become obsolete. The volume of literature available to nurses is too large to stay continually up to date, and transferring this research evidence into practice is sometimes difficult. For a nursing student, finding the best evidence for practice may seem daunting.

Fortunately a lot of research has already been conducted, systematically reviewed and critically appraised. Websites such as that of the Joanna Briggs Institute, among others, provide research for practice in an easy-to-understand format called systematic reviews and best-practice information sheets. These documents provide a summary of the best available evidence. Ask your librarian for advice about the best websites for accessing this type of quality research information.

Something to think about...

Every time you undertake nursing care or make a clinical decision, your action is based on something. It maybe something that you have heard or read, or what your intuition tells you is the right thing to do. It is your professional responsibility to ask: 'How do I know that this is really the most accurate decision or action?' Some practices that are based on information other than research are simply not the best way of doing things.

Coaching tips

Consider some of the procedures that you perform on a clinical placement. Where did the knowledge on which you base your practice come from? Are you sure that your knowledge and practice are evidence-based?

Activity

Select one of the skills you've learnt and practised on clinical placement. Access the Joanna Briggs Institute website or another similar site and review your knowledge and practice in light of the best available evidence. Ask yourself 'What are you doing? Why are you doing it? Why are you doing it that way? Is there a better way? What is the best way?' As a starting point, look at the following websites:

<http://www.joannabriggs.edu.au/about/home.php>
<http://www.cochrane.org>

Tips and tales 3.10
Practice principles

The performance of any nursing skill or procedure is informed by guiding practice principles. From these principles, behaviours can be generated for each nursing skill. The integration of knowledge (theories, concepts, rationales, evidence) within each practice principle forms the foundation of the behaviours for the nursing skill. You can use practice principles as a tool to reflect critically upon your nursing. A set of behaviours for each nursing skill (for example, showering, wound care, assessment of vital signs) can be generated using practice principles.

Table 3.1 identifies a core set of principles that applies to any nursing skill undertaken.

Table 3.1 Practice principles

Guiding practice principle	Examples of behaviours undertaken and informed from practice principles	Knowledge (e.g. theories, concepts, rationales, evidence)
Establishment of a need	• Assessment of health status • Monitoring changes in the patient • Implementing patient treatment orders (i.e. medication is due)	• Normal health status • Anatomy and physiology • Pharmacokinetics • Medication administration
Establishment of a state of readiness for nurse, patient and equipment	• Explanation to the patient • Checking to make sure the patient has time for the procedure (i.e. patient is not scheduled for an X-ray) • Collection of equipment required • The nurse identifies that the necessary support is available for the procedure (i.e. personnel to help with positioning or to check medications)	• Communication • Time management • Understanding hospital processes • Knowledge about resources and equipment necessary for undertaking the procedure
Maintenance of patient safety and comfort	• Hand-washing technique (social and/or surgical washes) • Providing pain relief before the start of a procedure • Positioning the patient before undertaking the procedure	• Asepsis • Microorganisms • Pain • Pharmacology • Body alignment
Prevention of untoward outcomes	• Providing assistance to the patient as necessary • Ending the procedure (removal of rubbish to prevent cross-infection)	• Respect • Cross-infection

Continued

Table 3.1 Practice principles *(continued)*

Guiding practice principle	Examples of behaviours undertaken and informed from practice principles	Knowledge (e.g. theories, concepts, rationales, evidence)
Assessment of patient's participation	• Assessing and/or encouraging the patient to participate • Encouraging self-care • Providing patient education to promote patient participation in health goals	• Motivation • Assessment of health • Self-care • Patient education • Health • Goal setting • Ethics
Evaluation of the activity in terms of effectiveness and appropriateness	• Assessment of patient and monitoring changes during and following the procedure (e.g. side effects of drugs) • Evaluation of patient (e.g. comfort)	• Assessment • Health status • Normal structure and function • Pharmacology • Comfort • Caring
Accuracy of reporting and recording	Reporting outcomes (i.e. handover report) Recording data and procedure undertaken (i.e. nursing notes)	• Reporting • Recording • Legal considerations • Communication

Adapted from Andersen 1991

Activity

1. Select one nursing procedure you are familiar with (e.g. temperature measurement, blood pressure measurement, showering a patient). Beside each guiding principle in Table 3.1 list the behaviours that you would undertake to competently perform the selected procedure. Be specific in describing your actions. To facilitate your learning, cross-check your behaviours with a basic or fundamental nursing text that describes nursing skills (Crisp & Taylor 2005).

2. Consider the behaviours associated with each principle for your selected nursing skill. Develop a list of learning issues (knowledge, concepts, research, theories, rationales etc) for follow-up that will allow you to expand your knowledge associated with the selected skill.

Tips and tales 3.11
Clinical governance

Clinical governance is a framework designed to help clinicians improve quality and safeguard standards of care. It is a fundamental principle that encourages openness about strengths and weaknesses, and incorporates the need to be proactive in order to improve through best practice (Duffy & Irvine 2004; Greco et al 2004). Clinical governance requires accountability and responsibility for quality care (Tait 2004). Clinical governance is about having the right people, policies, processes and information to be effective in delivering healthcare.

Many quality improvement strategies are implemented in the clinical environment. You may be involved in strategies such as risk management, audits and staff development, where clinical governance frameworks are used as a coordinating mechanism for quality.

The guiding principles of clinical governance include (Tait 2004):

- a focus on continuous quality improvement
- application to all facets of health care, across all service areas, models of practice, and inclusive of all healthcare providers through teamwork and sharing
- development of partnerships between all people involved (patients and their families, managers, clinicians, students)
- involvement of patients and the public
- learning from mistakes
- openness about failure

- emphasis on learning
- development of a just culture where individuals are treated fairly

During clinical placements you will find evidence of clinical governance principles being implemented and will certainly be involved in different strategies. Each institution will interpret the principles differently and will implement strategies that have meaning and relevance to patients, the community and staff in that facility. For example, there may be systems and infrastructure implemented to ensure quality of care, a set of guidelines or standards that you will be required to use, and mechanisms for data collection so that analysis and reports about care provision and services can be generated. In some cases these reports are directly linked to funding for the institution.

Some examples of clinical governance include the following (Duffy & Irvine 2004; Sydney West Area Health Service 2006; Tait 2004):

- management of serious complaints
- performance reviews
- clinical audits
- management of incidents and accidents
- critical incident review
- clinical practice improvement programs (for example, care pathways, standard setting)
- education, training and staff development programs
- accreditation and external quality reviews
- benchmarking processes
- policy generation

Coaching tips

- Understand the principles of clinical governance.
- Discuss with members of the interdisciplinary team their understanding of clinical governance principles and how the

principles contribute to sharing information and care provision with this framework.

- Actively contribute to strategies that support clinical governance frameworks.
- Reflect upon the shared beliefs and values of the interdisciplinary team. Analyse these in regard to the culture of the clinical learning environment.
- Identify the systems and tools that have been implemented to facilitate quality of care. Question others about how these systems have changed and improved practice (for example, an imprest system for stock management, an appraisal system, feedback mechanisms, case management reviews, and education sessions).
- Continually re-evaluate your own practice through reference to standards, evidence-based practice, policy and legislation.

Tips and tales 3.12
Clinical learning objectives

When on a clinical placement your learning will be both opportunistic and structured. In this section we'll talk about how clinical objectives help to provide structure and direction to your learning experience. In some ways a set of clinical objectives is like a well thought out itinerary. It guides your clinical journey, keeps you focused on the most important areas and can be used to communicate to others (for example, clinical educators and mentors) what you hope to achieve and where your interests lie. Your clinical objectives may be prescribed or you may be required to develop your own. Either way they should be SMART (Fowler 1998):

S	Specific
M	Measurable
A	Achievable
R	Realistic
T	Timely

Learning objectives help you become a safe, effective, competent and confident registered nurse. Your objectives will become progressively more sophisticated as you proceed through your program and each semester they will build upon and consolidate what you have already learnt.

Coaching tips

When developing your clinical learning objectives you should consider the following questions:

- What do you want to learn (objective)?
- Why do you want to learn it (rationale)?
- How are you going to learn it (strategy)?
- How are you going to prove that you have achieved your objective (evidence)?

An example of a clinical objective

Objective: To become competent and confident in assessing patients' blood pressure and determining whether it falls within normal parameters for the individual.

Rationale: Assessing blood pressure is a vital nursing skill and an important indication of a patient's haemodynamic and cardiovascular status. This is a skill that I do not feel confident with.

Strategy: I will research best practice guidelines regarding blood pressure assessment, practise the skill in the clinical laboratory at university and on placement, and ask for feedback from my mentor and educator.

Evidence: When I feel competent and confident I will ask my clinical educator to complete the blood pressure skills assessment form to confirm my achievement of this objective.

Developing learning objectives will require you to reflect upon your previous clinical experiences and review your strengths and limitations. Read sections 4.2 (Reflective practice) and 4.3 (Reality check and seeking feedback) before you begin to develop your objectives. You will also need to be self-directed and insightful in order to develop objectives that are meaningful and relevant to your stage of development. Use the ANMC Competency Standard for the Registered Nurse as a benchmark to help you analyse what you already know and can do, and where you need to focus, consolidate, develop and improve. Also consider the context of your placement and your scope of practice (review section 1.6, Working within your scope of practice). There is no point in having the objective 'develop knowledge and skills in the management of a central line' if you are a first-year student about to begin a placement in an aged care facility. Remember also that your clinical objectives should focus on the development of knowledge, skills *and* attitudes.

Finally, it is wise to discuss your objectives with your clinical educator or mentor, who will be able to determine if your objectives meet the SMART criteria listed above. It is important to know early on in a placement whether or not your objectives are realistic for your level of experience, and if you'll be able to achieve your objectives in a particular unit, with a particular patient mix, and within a specific time frame. Don't be surprised if your objectives need to be amended slightly.

Tips and tales 3.13
Student assessment

The clinical learning environment is an important component of formal learning, and assessment of student clinical performance forms an essential part of the teaching–learning process (Santy & Mackintosh 2000; Watson et al 2002). Assessment allows you to gain a sense of achievement, to gauge your progress and to appreciate your ability to practice in the real world.

Various forms of clinical assessments are used in practice. Some assessments are designed to provide you with ongoing feedback, others determine your competence (perhaps in performing a nursing skill), and some may provide a measure of your skills or knowledge based on a set of criteria (Fisher & Parolin 2000; Goldsmith et al 2006; Watson et al 2002). The Australian National Competency Standards (ANMC 2005) underlie many assessments related to clinical (and on-campus) performance. For example, you may be required to complete an appraisal of your performance (that is, a self-assessment) before your mentor assesses you, based on the competency standards. Other examples of clinical assessments may include the following:

- You may be required to undertake patient transfer techniques with your clinical educator, who will complete a feedback sheet that becomes a critical element for your portfolio submission. A self-assessment of your transfer technique may also be needed for the portfolio.
- You might be asked to attend to a set of nursing care procedures under supervision, which may then be rated according to best-practice guidelines.
- Alternatively, you may be expected to collect data that will form the basis of an assessment item, such as the direct observation of wound healing.

For some assessments, your institution may state that you must be assessed by people who are qualified to assess you (that is, your clinical educator or an appropriately approved assessor). For other assessments, it may be that the person you are working with (your mentor) would be the most appropriate person to assess you.

Self-assessment of your clinical performance is also a valuable learning tool. Different approaches to self-assessment based on the ANMC standards (2005) are used in nursing programs across Australia and professionally. This form of assessment helps you prepare for clinical placement. When you inform your supervisors of your learning objectives at the beginning of the placement, you could include assessments and practice requests. Providing evidence of self-assessment before the placement demonstrates the preparation you have done and facilitates early opportunities to undertake assessments. Remember that care requirements for patients are always paramount and your need to complete an assessment must not compromise the health or welfare of a patient. You should also be considerate of staff workloads and other pressures (Edmond 2001).

There are many competing needs in a clinical learning environment and you should focus on the broader picture rather than your personal needs. On some placements there may be situations or issues that make it difficult for you to undertake your required assessments. Examples of these could include:

- There are limited opportunities in the clinical learning environment to allow you to undertake the assessment.
- The supervisor is unable to assess you because of the competing demands of others (for example, patient care demands or other students).
- The number of student assessments to be undertaken does not allow all students the opportunity for practice or supervision.
- Some students require more supervision than others and these students take more of the supervisor's time. There is an inequitable time given to all students for supervision.
- Students are too slow because they have not taken the time to practise the procedures before their clinical placement. The assessor deems that the student is not ready to be assessed at the time of request.

Coaching tips

- Discuss assessment requirements with supervisors early in the placement. You may find that making an appointment with a supervisor facilitates processes and relieves pending anxiety.

- Communicate any difficulties you perceive about meeting the assessment requirements to the appropriate person (this may be the clinical educator, lecturer or registered nurse) as soon as you identify them.
- As with all nursing care, the principles of safe practice must be integrated into your assessment.
- Know and use the ANMC standards (2005) to inform your practice.
- Take advantage of practice opportunities on campus (such as laboratory sessions) to ensure that you are ready for assessment and related care requirements. Self-assess your performance during these sessions using the statements and cues from the ANMC standards.
- Identify competing needs, organisational, clinical, educational or practical.

Tips and tales 3.14
Giving and receiving gifts

In this section we focus on giving and receiving gifts, which has the potential to be a boundary violation for nurses (see section 4.6 for a general discussion of boundary violations). While society views gift giving as a normal occurrence to show appreciation, giving or receiving gifts in the context of the nurse–patient therapeutic relationship has the potential to invoke emotional discomfort and embarrassment, and to compromise a relationship where trust, rapport and the power balance may be open to exploitation.

Patients often express their gratitude by giving a small gift at the end of their stay as a gesture of thanks. This type of gift is usually given to one nurse but is accepted on behalf of the team. It may take the form of tokens such as flowers, chocolates or fruit, which are left at the nurses' station for sharing. Boundary violations can be avoided by declining a personal gift and accepting the gift on behalf of the team.

Assess the appropriateness of any gift that is offered to ensure that you do not violate your professional boundaries. There are several factors to consider when a gift is offered (Nurses Registration Board New South Wales 1999):

- the timing of the gift in relation to the patient care episode (before, during, after care is provided)
- the intent of the gift and any expectation of different care being provided as a result of the gift
- the potential consequences of accepting or refusing the gift, such as family responses or any emotional discomfort

Consider the following story.

Linda had been caring for Mrs Fairford, an elderly woman, for several weeks when suddenly her patient gave her a pair of earrings that she had owned since she was 18 years old. She stated that she wanted Linda to have them because she didn't think she would be still be around the following week when Linda returned to placement. Linda assured Mrs Fairford that she would see her the following week and at first refused the gift. When Mrs Fairford reasserted her desire for Linda to have them Linda finally accepted.

Mrs Fairford passed away during Linda's days off and when her family came to collect her belongings they noticed that their mother's earrings were missing. The family demanded that the earrings be found. The patient's room was thoroughly searched, but of course the earrings were not found. The nursing unit manager asked to speak to all staff who had cared for Mrs Fairford. It was at this interview that Linda found out that the earrings she had been given by Mrs Fairford had been reported missing by the family. Mrs Fairford had not informed her family of her decision to give Linda the earrings, nor had Linda told anyone about her gift.

What are your thoughts about this situation? Was it appropriate for Linda to have accepted the gift? Did Linda violate a principle of professional practice? What impact did this gift have on the family and on Linda?

Coaching tips

- Consider carefully whether you should accept a gift offered by a patient.
- If you do accept a token gift, accept it on behalf of the team.
- Seek advice from your mentor or nursing unit manager about a gift that is offered by a patient or a patient's family member.

Another perspective to consider is the giving of gifts by nursing students. Students sometimes feel that they would like to show their appreciation to staff who have been involved in their learning. When giving a gift be mindful that you do not place a colleague or supervisor in a position where they feel pressured or uncomfortable.

Usually, the best way to offer a gift is as a parting gesture. It may be more appropriate if the gift is offered by a group rather than an individual (this of course depends on the number of students allocated to the clinical educator or unit). Here are some suggestions for ways to show appreciation:

- Verbal thanks can be expressed directly to your mentor and to the manager of the unit.
- A card or certificate expressing your appreciation can be given. Be specific—name the people who went out of their way for you and say what you gained from your experience.
- A gift such as a pot plant, flowers, a basket of fruit or box of chocolates is always appreciated.
- Some of our students have provided morning tea for the staff on the last day of their placement.

Accepting thanks

It is equally important to accept appreciation from the nursing staff for your contribution. I recently overheard a registered nurse thanking a student for her hard work and telling her that her clinical skills were outstanding. The student's response was to downplay and minimise her success: 'It was nothing', she shyly replied. Minimising words are those that diminish or deprecate the importance of your achievement. While nurses may not have cornered the market in the use of minimising words, they certainly use them too often.

- Practise responding to compliments and thanks positively: for example, 'Thank you, it was my pleasure'.
- Don't use words such as 'I only…', 'It was nothing' or 'I just…'.
- If you must be modest, try saying, 'Thank you, I'm pleased with my progress. I really did have a lot of support and guidance from the registered nurses I worked with here'.

Tips and tales 3.15
Documentation and legal issues

Quality documentation is a requirement of all healthcare professionals. Documentation may make or break the defence of a hospital and staff if legal action is instigated following a critical incident or unexplained death. Currently Australia has one of the highest incidences of medical litigation in the developed world.

Some points to consider

- Documentation is considered to be the most important evidence in a potential legal action and therefore its significance should never be underestimated.

- Legal action may be initiated many years after a critical incident occurs. Memories of witnesses will obviously fade and therefore accurate documentation may be crucial to the outcome of the case.
- Accurate documentation will ensure that your nursing report demonstrates evidence of the care given to your patients, as well as providing a means of communication between health professionals.
- Accurate documentation means more relevant documentation, not more extensive documentation.
- Quality documentation will save you time and may protect you from potential litigation.
- Remember the best answer to litigation is concise, accurate, objective and contemporaneous documentation.

Coaching tips

- Reports should be concise. Avoid verbosity and 'double charting'. Document only aberrations from normal in the integrated progress notes. Avoid useless and unnecessarily long words and sentences. Use care plans and clinical pathways as adjuncts to integrated progress notes, but do not duplicate information.
- Reports should be accurate. You should distinguish between what you personally observe and what is related to you by another person (hearsay): for example, 'The patient stated that she had slipped over', not 'The patient slipped over'. Unless you have actually witnessed the incident, the patient's complaint is hearsay and must be reported as such.
- Reports should be objective. Avoid using the word 'appears'. You should record what you actually see, not what you think you see: for example, 'The patient appears to be in shock' should instead be documented as 'The patient is pale and sweating,

hypotensive, BP 80/40, tachycardic, pulse 140, with peripheral cyanosis', or 'The patient was observed at two-hourly intervals during the night, and when so observed was sleeping', not 'Patient appears to have slept all night'.

- Documentation should be contemporaneous. It should be written as close as possible to the time when the incident or treatment occurred. Memories fade and often one incident is followed closely by a series of incidents, particularly if a patient's condition deteriorates and a number of treatments are initiated. Trying to put this in sequence at the end of the shift can be confusing and lead to inaccuracies.
- Always sign and print your name, and include your designation and educational institution at the end of your report.
- Documentation should be specific. Say exactly what you mean: for example, 'Patient experienced a sudden onset of severe breathlessness following ambulation, respiratory rate 40', not 'Patient feeling breathless'.
- Documentation should be legible, with correct spelling and grammar. Nurses often complain about doctors' handwriting, but they too may be at fault. If a negligence case is taken to court, your nursing notes may be used as evidence. Imagine how you'd feel if your notes could not be interpreted because of poor legibility. Furthermore, reports filled with misspelt words and incorrect grammar create the same negative impression as illegible handwriting.
- Document all relevant information. Document any change in the patient's condition, what you observed to support this observation, your follow-up actions and whom you notified of the change. Also document if there has been no change in the patient's condition during your shift. Do not document normal observations that have been charted elsewhere, such as vital signs, postoperative observations and voiding or drain patency, but do document if there are any aberrations from normal

and what your actions were. The use of clinical pathways and care plans has significantly reduced the need for extensive documentation in the integrated progress notes.

- Only accepted abbreviations are to be used. Nurses work in many different institutions during their clinical placements and later employment. A diversity of abbreviations can lead to confusing and misleading interpretations: for example, the abbreviation SB can be taken to mean 'short of breath' or 'seen by'. Make sure you understand the meaning of any medical and nursing abbreviations used and include only commonly accepted and easy-to-understand abbreviations in your notes.

- An error should be dealt with by drawing a line through the incorrect entry and initialling it. Total obliteration may suggest that you have something to hide. White-out should not be used for the same reason.

- Never make an entry in a patient's notes before checking the name and medical record number (MRN) on the patient's chart. Don't rely on room numbers only. Patients are often moved from room to room, and have also been known to 'get into the wrong bed'.

- All omissions should be documented. If you do not carry out an ordered treatment or procedure, always document why it was omitted and who you notified. If nothing is written, it may be presumed that the procedure was overlooked. For example, if a patient's hypertensive medication was not administered because the patient's blood pressure was too low, this must be documented in the patient's notes and the medication chart. The follow-up action and the person notified should be included. When you are busy with patient care, documentation may seem to be of secondary importance. However, from a coroner's point of view an incomplete chart may suggest incomplete nursing care. This is not always true, but it is an easy inference to make. You may have performed a nursing procedure and you simply forgot to chart it, but if a dispute arises many years later you will have nothing to back up your version of the facts, assuming you can even remember what you did at the time.

- Be aware that the assumption is made that if something is not documented then it has not been done.
- Never make an entry in a patient's notes of behalf of another person.
- Be aware that nurses are practising in an era of consumerism. This has created a more litigious and complaint-oriented society. In order to protect themselves from potential litigation, nurses need higher-quality and more relevant documentation. They should always bear in mind that they will be held accountable for the care provided to patients and may be called upon to explain their actions in relation to patient care. Good-quality documentation is part of a nurses' accountability and may be the only assistance nurses can rely upon if asked to explain their professional actions.

Tips and tales 3.16
Visitors during clinical placements

Clinical placements require a field agreement or a memorandum of understanding. These agreements between the educational institution and the healthcare facility set out requirements, restrictions and conditions for the placement. Students are therefore bound by specific rules, regulations and policies. As a general principle, students are not to receive personal visitors during clinical placement. However, if a personal visit is anticipated, you should discuss it in advance with the appropriate person. Facilities have in place policies that guide special circumstances, such as the needs of breastfeeding mothers.

Coaching tips

- Inform your family and friends that it is inappropriate for them to visit you on clinical placement unless it is an emergency.
- Instruct family members about how to contact you in an emergency. Document your placement details (facility, shift, ward and contact number) for urgent contact requirements.
- Ensure that your contact details are current on your educational institution database system (especially emergency contact details).
- If you have unwanted visitors while on clinical placement, immediately seek assistance from the nursing unit manager and/or facility security. Contact your clinical educator for assistance and advice.

Tips and tales 3.17
Using the company supplies

Nursing students undertaking clinical placements enter health facilities where resources are calculated and costed for patient care. Those students who help themselves to health facility supplies contribute to costs associated with the health budget.

You should also consider what is provided by the facility for staff and what they themselves contribute. Consider the following story.

Cathy's clinical placement was in a small private clinic. On orientation to the facility, the nurse unit manager showed Cathy the staff tearoom, but requested that she go to the cafeteria in the next building for all her meal breaks. On the second day of the placement, Cathy decided that she couldn't be bothered walking to the cafeteria and helped herself to coffee and biscuits in the staff tearoom. The staff said nothing about her using the tearoom and she continued to have her meal breaks in the staff tearoom for the rest of her placement. Cathy was not aware that some of the staff were annoyed about her using their facilities. She did not know that the tearoom supplies were purchased from a staff fund.

Not all facilities provide supplies for staff tearooms. While a cafeteria may be available for staff use, the staff may contribute to a social club for personal items to support their working environment. These purchases may include the following:

- tea, coffee, biscuits, milk, sugar and juice
- filtered water cooler
- fruit basket supply
- lunch provisions (bread, butter, spreads etc)
- soap and shampoo for showers
- subscriptions to newspapers, magazines, journals

You should not assume that food, drink and supplies left in a common tearoom are available for your use.

Apart from tearoom supplies there are other resources you should think about before helping yourself. For example, letterhead stationary is expensive and students should not use it as notepaper. Neither should you use preprinted forms (such as medication charts or observation forms) for this purpose.

Similarly, you should ask permission to use the ward photocopier. Think about what it is you are copying, whether you can access the information somewhere else (for instance, from your own computer through internet links, or from a library) and the amount of paper that may be used. Also be mindful of copyright laws. Photocopying is calculated and contributes to the ward or unit budget.

It should not have to be said, but for those that are unsure the health facility is not a place to access supplies for your first aid kit. Removal of supplies from a facility without permission constitutes theft. Similarly, newspapers and magazines should be left for patients and visitors to read.

Coaching tips

- Be organised for your clinical placement by ensuring that you take essential equipment with you (notebook, pens, safety equipment etc).
- Have a notebook (the size of your pocket) to document important notes (remember to adhere to privacy issues).
- Be prepared to contribute to a ward social fund, especially if you are on a ward or unit for an extended period of time.

Reflective thinking activities

What advice would you give the student in the following scenario?

One of your fellow nursing students is undertaking a six-week clinical placement in intensive care. She confides in you that the husband of an unconscious patient she has been caring for is making her feel very uncomfortable. At first he told her what a lovely, caring nurse she was, and then he began to ask her questions about her personal life—where she lived, if she had a boyfriend, and so on. In the beginning she thought he was just being friendly, but lately he has been standing too close to her when she is caring for his wife, and touching her as she walks past him. She mentioned her discomfort to one of the registered nurses she was working with, but he brushed it off, saying that the man 'probably didn't mean any harm'.

What would you do in the following situation?

It is the first day of your second-year clinical placement. You are sitting in the tearoom with some of the nursing staff when another student walks in and asks a question about one of the patients she is caring for.

The staff answer her question somewhat impatiently but when she walks out a few of them begin singing 'Bring in the clowns...'. Laughingly they tell you that they are really tired of the silly questions the other student keeps asking.

References

Andersen BM 1991 Mapping the terrain of the discipline. In G. Gray & R. Pratt (eds), Towards a discipline of nursing, pp 95–123. Churchill Livingstone, Melbourne.

Ang I, Brand JE, Noble G & Wilding D 2002 Living diversity. Australia's multicultural future. Special Broadcasting Service Artarmon, Sydney.

ANMC 2005 ANMC National Competency Standards for the Registered Nurse. Australian Nursing and Midwifery Council, Canberra.

Chaska N 2000 The nursing profession: tomorrow and beyond. Sage, Thousand Oaks.

Crisp J & Taylor C (eds) 2005 Potter and Perry's fundamentals of nursing, 2nd edn. Mosby, Sydney.

Dawes M, Davies P, Gray A et al 2005 A primer for health care professionals. Elsevier, Edinburgh.

Duffy E 1995 Horizontal violence: a conundrum for nursing. Collegian 2(2):5–17.

Duffy JA & Irvine EA 2004 Clinical governance: a system. Quality in Primary Care 12:141–145.

Edmond CB 2001 A new paradigm for practice education. Nurse Education Today 21:251–259.

Farrell G 1997 Aggression in clinical settings: nurses' views. Journal of Advanced Nursing 25:501–508.

Fisher M & Parolin M 2000 The reliability of measuring clinical performance using a competency based assessment tool: a pilot study. Collegian 7(3):21–27.

Fowler J (ed) 1998 The handbook of clinical supervision—your questions answered. Quay Books, Salisbury.

Gardner S & Johnson P 2001 Sexual harassment in healthcare: strategies for employers. Hospital Topics 79(4):5–11.

Goldsmith M, Stewart L & Ferguson L 2006 Peer learning partnership: an innovative strategy to enhance skill acquisition in nursing students. Nurse Education Today 26(2):123–130.

Greco M, Powell R, Jolliffe J et al 2004 Evaluation of a clinical governance training programme for non-executive directors of NHS organisations. Quality in Primary Care 12:119–127.

Griffin M 2004 Teaching cognitive rehearsal as a shield for lateral violence: an intervention for newly licensed nurses. Journal of Continuing Education in Nursing 35(6):257–264.

Hamlin L & Hoffman A 2002 Perioperative nurses and sexual harassment. AORN Journal 76(5):855–860.

Joanna Briggs Institute 2004 Levels of evidence. Online. Available <www.joannabriggs.edu.au/pubs/approach.php?mde+TEXT>, 1 May 2005.

Kikuchi JF 2005 Cultural theories of nursing responsive to human needs and values. Journal of Nursing Scholarship 37(4):302–307.

Leininger MM 1991 The theory of culture care diversity and universality. In MM Leininger (ed.), Culture care diversity & universality: a theory of nursing, pp 5–68. National League for Nursing, New York.

Madison J & Minichicello V 2001 Sexual harassment in healthcare— classification of harassers and rationalizations of sex based harassment behavior. Journal of Nursing Administration 3(11):534–543.

Millenson ML 1997 Demanding medical evidence. University of Chicago Press, Chicago.

Nurses Registration Board New South Wales 1999 A project report to the Nurses Registration Board of New South Wales on the development of guidelines for registered nurses and enrolled nurses regarding the boundaries of practice. Online. Available <www.nmb.nsw.gov.au/Boundaries-of-Professional-Practice/default.aspx>, 16 April 2004.

Santy J & Mackintosh C 2000 Assessment and learning in post-registration nurse education. Nursing Standard 14(18):38–41.

Schim S, Doorenbos A & Borse N 2005 Cultural competence among Ontario and Michigan healthcare providers. Journal of Nursing Scholarship 37(4):354–360.

Stark MA, Manning-Walsh J & Vliem S 2005 Caring for self while learning to care for others: a challenge for nursing students. Journal of Nursing Education 44(6):266–270.

Sydney West Area Health Service 2006 Clinical governance. Online. Available <http://www.wsahs.nsw.gov.au/services/clinicalgovernance/index.htm>, 13 January 2006.

Tait AR 2004 Clinical governance in primary care: a literature review. Issues in Clinical Nursing 13:723–730.

Thompson IE, Melia KM & Boyd KM 2000 Nursing ethics. Churchill Livingstone, Edinburgh.

Watson R, Stimpson A, Topping A et al 2002 Clinical competence assessment in nursing: a systematic review of the literature. Journal of Advanced Nursing 39(5):421–431.

Chapter 4

How you think and feel

If one learns from others but does not think, one will be bewildered. If, on the other hand, one thinks but does not learn from others, one will be in peril.

Confucius (551–479 BC), Chinese philosopher

Tips and tales 4.1
Caring

Nurses enter the nursing profession because they care about people and society. However, nurses don't have the monopoly on caring. Parents care for their children; teachers care about their students; doctors provide clinical care for their patients; chaplains provide pastoral care. So why do professionals view caring differently? Caring is one of those concepts that can be elusive and have different meanings. The literature provides many examples, definitions and theories of caring (Walsh & Walsh 1999; Watson et al 2002; Williams 1998). For some, caring and nursing may seem to be the same, but others will differentiate caring from nursing.

Nurses understand caring from many perspectives that reflect their experiences, context of practice and knowledge. One way to understand caring would be to view it as discourses of caring. Discourses are groups of statements that act to constrain and enable what we know (Bourgeois 2006). A finite number of statements contribute to a discourse and these recur time and again, so that we come to see certain statements (often made by very prominent people) as truths. Take for example the statement, 'Caring is nursing'. This often-repeated statement in the literature is perceived differently by individual nurses.

Three discourses of caring are evident in nursing (Bourgeois 2006)—that is, nurses speak about caring from a position within different discourses, using statements that define and inform others about caring. These discourses are 'caring as being', 'caring as doing' and 'caring as knowing'. Nurses who speak about caring will use statements that belong to these different discourses.

In the discourse 'caring as being', nurses speak about caring as an element that is intrinsic and essential for nurses. Caring for them is part of their nature as human beings, involving them in caring relationships. You may hear some of your peers claim, 'I was born to be a nurse. It is in my family; all my family are nurses', 'Caring is a part of me', or 'All I want is to do is care for others'.

The discourse 'caring as doing' is evident when nurses talk about caring as actions and behaviours. They may mention skills and procedures as proof of their caring actions for patients. Nurses speaking from within this discourse refer to caring using complex concepts such as providing comfort, showing compassion and helping others.

'Caring as knowing' is a discourse that contributes ideas and practices associated with the knowledge base essential for nursing. Nurses use statements in which they claim to own caring. Caring theorists have contributed much to this discourse (Leininger 1991; Orem 1991; Watson 1999; Watson et al 2002).

Consider the following questions:

- Nursing is often called the caring profession. Is this how you view nursing?
- When observing the nurses you work with, what elements of their practice would you identify as caring and why?
- What would constitute uncaring practices by nurses?

Coaching tips

- Reflect on the meaning of caring and identify what it means to you. Try to define caring. Identify how you demonstrate caring in your practice. Seek feedback about your practice from patients, peers and mentors. Does this feedback support your definitions and ideas about what caring is?
- Consider practices that may affect your placement and your ability to undertake care: for example, the mix of staff on the ward or the model of care implemented.
- Compare your nursing practice with that of others. What similarities and differences are there?

- Consider your personality, philosophy and beliefs. How do these affect your caring practices?
- Consider the different types of placements you undertake throughout your program. Do you care differently for patients in different practice contexts? Compare, for example, caring for people in a perioperative, emergency room or aged care placement.
- Ask your patients for feedback about your practice. Ask specific questions: do they feel that you give them enough time, that you listen to them, and that you undertake nursing care in a timely manner?

Tips and tales 4.2
Reflective practice

Something to think about...

Learning without thought is labour lost; thought without learning is perilous.
Confucius (Chinese philosopher, 551–479 BC)

At the risk of stating the obvious, simply undertaking a clinical placement does not necessarily develop competence—just being there does not guarantee learning. Developing competency involves not only taking action in practice but also learning from practice through reflection. Reflection is intrinsic to learning. It allows nurses to process their experience, explore their understanding of what they are doing, why they are doing it, and what impact it has on themselves and others (Boud 1999).

The skill of reflection is pivotal to the development of your clinical knowledge and understanding. Reflection allows you to consider your personal and professional skills and to identify needs for ongoing development. As a student nurse you should become increasingly aware of your professional values, skills, strengths and areas that require further development.

While we can and do learn from a wide range of experiences (good and bad) learning is often initiated by painful, difficult, embarrassing or uncomfortable experiences. Don't just try to forget about these challenging times. Reflection is about exploration, questioning, learning and growing through, and as a consequence of, these experiences.

Devoting some time to reflection during and after each clinical placement will allow you to plan for future clinical experiences and to develop clear and appropriate objectives for your next placement. At the very least, reflecting on your experience provides information that you can take to clinical or academic staff for help or guidance in further skill development.

Keeping a journal

The process of reflection provides the raw data of experiences. In order to use these experiences creatively, to transform them into knowledge, the additional stage of writing is required. Writing fixes thoughts on paper. As you stare at the paper, and stare at what you have written, your objectified thinking stares back at you. As you rearrange your writings, you often find that you are loosening your imagination by combining various ideas and thoughts. Creative ideas occur during the mechanical process of giving them shape (van Manen 1990). Reflections are the raw materials, but they are turned into knowledge as you write—sometimes you don't know how much you know until you write it down.

Many nursing programs require students to participate in some form of formal written reflection. Students often have to submit a journal describing their reflections about their clinical experience, including application of relevant theory, and their understanding of their experience. Even if this is not a formal requirement at your educational institution, it is certainly wise to keep a personal journal as the reflective writing process allows you to clarify your values, affirm your strengths and identify your learning needs.

Discerning and describing the knowledge, competence and skills that go into day-to-day nursing work allow nurses to understand their work in a more empowering way. This increases nurses' mastery and appreciation of their own work and their ability to better care for patients (Buresh & Gordon 2000).

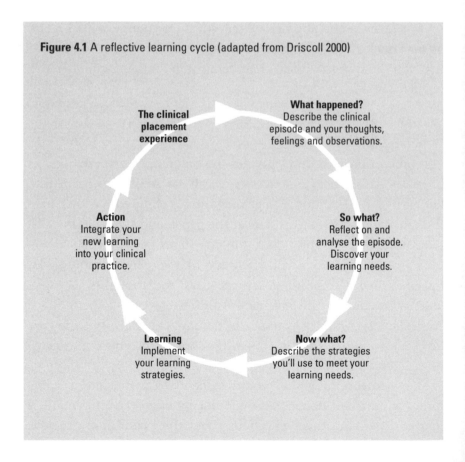

Figure 4.1 A reflective learning cycle (adapted from Driscoll 2000)

The clinical placement experience

What happened?
Describe the clinical episode and your thoughts, feelings and observations.

So what?
Reflect on and analyse the episode. Discover your learning needs.

Now what?
Describe the strategies you'll use to meet your learning needs.

Learning
Implement your learning strategies.

Action
Integrate your new learning into your clinical practice.

Something to think about...

Observation tells us the fact, reflection the meaning of the fact.
Florence Nightingale (in Baly 1991)

Coaching tips

There are many resources to help you develop your ability to become a reflective practitioner, and your lecturers may recommend a process. Figure 4.1 is a diagrammatic representation of one method of reflection that many students find clear and easy to follow. Give it a try—you may be surprised how insightful you become! Then read Mr Jackson's story.

Mr Jackson's story is an example of reflective journal writing and the application of the ANMC competency standards (2005). Behaviours that reflect an element of the ANMC competencies are highlighted in bold text and the relevant competency is given in square brackets.

---

*I was looking after Mr Jackson (pseudonym), a 76-year-old man, who was 2 days post-op following a right hip replacement. As I entered Mr Jackson's room to take his 10 a.m. observations **I noticed that he was restless** [5.2 Uses a range of assessment techniques to collect relevant and accurate data] and when I spoke to him he did not seem to comprehend my questions, replying inappropriately. **I did not recall his confusion being reported at handover. I introduced myself to Mr Jackson and his wife** [9.1 Establishes therapeutic relationships that are goal directed and recognises professional boundaries] and **asked whether Mr Jackson had been confused before his hospital admission** [5.2 Uses a range of assessment techniques to collect relevant and accurate data]. His wife replied that she had never seen him like this before.*

*I reassured her and explained [9.2 Communicates
effectively with individuals/groups to facilitate provision of care]* that
I would take his observations and then *consult the RN I was
working with [7.3 Prioritises workload based on the individual's/
group's needs, acuity and optimal time for intervention]. I realised
that this situation was beyond my scope of practice*
[2.5 Understands and practises within own scope of practice].

*I started to consider some of the possible causes for
Mr Jackson's confusion. I wondered whether he was in
pain* but he did not reply when I asked about his pain. I thought that
he might have been hypoxic, and when I took his SaO2 it was
80 per cent and his respiratory rate 28. His BP was elevated compared
to his preop BP; his pulse was rapid, full and bounding. He was
afebrile. *I checked that his IV was dripping and his catheter
draining. I also checked the wound dressing, which was
dry and intact [5.2 Uses a range of assessment techniques to collect
relevant and accurate data; 7.1 Effectively manages the nursing care
of individual/groups; 1.2 Fulfils the duty of care].*

I then documented my observations [1.1 Complies with
relevant legislation and common law]. *I reassured Mr Jackson
and his wife that I would consult with the RN and
return* [9.2 Communicates effectively with individual/groups to
facilitate provision of care]. *I put the bed rails up* [9.5 Facilitates
a physical, psychosocial, cultural and spiritual environment that
promotes individual/group safety and security] before I left the
room, as I was concerned for Mr Jackson's safety. *I discussed my
observations and concerns with the RN* [2.5 Understands
and practises within own scope of practice; 10.2 Communicates
nursing assessment and decisions to the interdisciplinary healthcare
team and other relevant service providers] who immediately returned
with me to review Mr Jackson.

The RN asked Mr Jackson to point to anywhere it hurt and he
touched his head. She checked the IV rate and found that it was

running at 125 mL hour. When the RN compared the rate to the fluid orders chart, she found it was meant to be running at 84 mL/hr. She calculated that the catheter had drained less than 40 mL in 4 hours. The RN asked Mr Jackson's wife if he was normally so puffy around his eyes and she replied that he wasn't. She listened to his chest with a stethoscope and rechecked his SaO2, this time with an ear probe as his hands were cold, which could give inaccurate results. The RN explained to Mr Jackson and his wife what she was doing and said that she would phone the doctor immediately.

Outside the room the RN explained to me that she suspected hypervolaemia, renal impairment and possibly electrolyte imbalance and that she was concerned that Mr Jackson would develop pulmonary oedema if he were not treated quickly. She thanked me for bringing Mr Jackson's cognitive impairment and abnormal observations to her attention. Review by the doctor and follow-up pathology tests later confirmed the RN's preliminarily nursing diagnosis.

*I feel that I undertook a good but very general assessment of Mr Jackson. However I realised after watching the RN that **I need to develop more focused and comprehensive assessment skills** [4.4 Uses appropriate strategies to manage own responses to the professional work environment]. I also believe that a deeper knowledge base would allow me to analyse and interpret abnormal observations more accurately. In particular, **I need an understanding of the potential causes of confusion in elderly patients, and skills and knowledge related to fluid status assessment so that I can provide a better standard of care to my patients** [3.1 Identifies the relevance of research to improving individual/group health outcomes; 4.2 Participates in professional development to enhance nursing practice]. It was inspiring to observe an RN who had the experience and knowledge to thoroughly and efficiently assess Mr Jackson and establish an accurate nursing diagnosis.*

Tips and tales 4.3
Reality check and seeking feedback

So far in this book we've focused on the clinical environment and your place in it. Now it's time to turn the focus completely onto you, by asking you to address the following questions:

- How do I see myself?
- How do others see me?

This is not a once-off activity, but rather a lifelong process of personal and professional development. This 'reality check' is pivotal to your ongoing growth and improvement and is a process that you'll find invaluable to your career success.

How do I see myself?

To answer this question you should begin by assessing and listing your skills and attributes (clinical, interpersonal and others) and identifying your strengths and limitations. Skills are acquired abilities. Attributes may be acquired or intrinsic. There are three main types of skills and attributes:

- technical or clinical skills, such as those involved in providing oral care to an unconscious patient or safely administering medications
- interpersonal skills, which include communication, empathy and being supportive (among others)
- personal attributes, such as adaptability, motivation, critical thinking and problem-solving

Take some time to reflect on your skills and consider areas in which you excel and those that require further development. Identifying gaps or limitations is just as important as acknowledging your strengths.

How do others see me?

Once you have completed your self-assessment, you should validate it by seeking feedback from others. You can obtain this feedback from managers, educators, clinicians and fellow students. Performance appraisals and informal feedback are invaluable to understanding how others perceive you. Asking for feedback is not always easy, but your success depends on your openness to different perspectives. It involves listening and accepting positive and negative feedback, and acknowledging the areas in which change and improvement are needed. Seeking advice about new skills that you require and strategies to develop them is also essential.

Now compare the skills and attributes that you identified with the feedback from others. Are there any discrepancies? Did others recognise skills and attributes that you were not aware of but can now build on? Were limitations identified that you were not aware of?

Something to think about...

If life is to have meaning, the extent to which you know yourself is the most important work that you will ever do. And because life is a process of emergence and becoming, it is a journey not a destination.
Crow 2000, p 33

Coaching tips

It is your right (and responsibility) as a student to seek ongoing and regular feedback about your performance. Most educational institutions have a formal process for ensuring this occurs. However, you should still seek informal feedback regularly. Ask for specific, concrete feedback about your skills, attributes, strengths and limitations and use the feedback as a springboard to success.

Lastly, receiving formal feedback should be a positive experience and should not display any hidden agendas, such as the discussion of any previously unmentioned problems. All problem areas—for example, poor time-management skills or unsafe practice—should be dealt with when they occur and not stored up to be revealed only at a performance review. You deserve regular formative feedback throughout your placement and opportunities to improve. Grievance procedures are available if disagreements are unable to be resolved between you and your assessor, and you should consult your educational policies for guidance. Conflict and confusion, if they arise, should be dealt with constructively and sensitively.

Tips and tales 4.4
Articulating your learning needs

Something to think about...

Nurses are so hesitant to ask for what they need, they cannot accept the idea of asking for what they want. It seems too self indulgent.
Chenevert 1985, p 116

In order to articulate your learning needs, you need to know what it is you require. A self-assessment is the key to exploring new opportunities (see section 4.3). It will assist you to develop a list of needs that can then be articulated to mentors, clinical teachers and healthcare team members so that learning opportunities can be enhanced.

The following story illustrates one student's dilemma and highlights a case where articulation of the learning student's needs would have helped her to achieve her goals.

Hui Fei was undertaking her final clinical placement. A component of this placement was her mentor's appraisal and sign-off on a set of clinical skills. On two occasions during the placement, Hui Fei's mentor asked her if she had any learning objectives that she needed help with. At no point did Hui Fei mention her appraisal or her sets of clinical skills, and told her mentor that she was OK.

At the end of her placement period, however, Hui Fei produced her book for sign-off. At this point her mentor said that she could not complete several elements of the appraisal and skill set because she had not observed and assessed Hui Fei's practice. Naturally Hui Fei became upset, because she could not complete the requirements. Her mentor pointed out that she had asked her on more than one occasion if there was anything she needed to complete, and emphasised she could not sign off on practices that she had not observed.

In this scenario, the student did not articulate her needs to the mentor early in the placement and on completion of the clinical placement the expectations of the mentor and student were not congruent. Effective communication strategies are essential so that you can express your learning needs. As a student you are encouraged to identify your learning needs early in the placement, re-evaluating them as necessary.

Coaching tips

- Be prepared for each clinical placement. Reflect on past experiences and your clinical strengths and weaknesses. Identify new learning appropriate for practice in the forthcoming placement environment.
- Find out about the opportunities available in the area of your clinical placement to determine your personal objectives (before your arrival on the first day).
- Introduce yourself to your clinical mentor. Discuss your learning objectives, assessment requirements, and scope of practice.

- Ask your mentor for strategies to help you achieve your learning objectives.
- Find a quiet place at an appropriate time to discuss your needs with your mentor.
- Remember that questions during patient care episodes disrupt the therapeutic relationship and remove the focus from the patient. Be respectful of the patient and the need for the nurse to concentrate.

Tips and tales 4.5
Ethical dilemmas in nursing

Something to think about ...

You should not decide until you have heard what both have to say.
Aristophanes (Greek playwright, c. 438 – c. 388 BC), *The Wasps*

What is ethics and why do nurses need to understand it?

Ethics, also known as morality, is often defined as the philosophical study of right or wrong action (Dahnke & Dreher 2006). This does not mean that ethics is of concern to philosophers alone. All human beings have pondered questions of right and wrong from time to time. It is essential for nurses to understand ethics, because in their day-to-day work they frequently encounter ethical questions and problems such as patient's rights, questions of life and death, and confidentiality. A clear understanding of ethics helps nurses interpret these difficult situations and to identify possible courses of action and the principles underpinning moral actions (Dahnke & Dreher 2006).

Ethical principles

Ethical principles are standards of conduct that make up an ethical system.

Autonomy. The ability to make free choices about oneself and one's life, to be self-governing. This principle is at the heart of informed consent.

Beneficence. To do good, and the obligation to act for the benefit of others.

Non-maleficence. To avoid doing harm.

Justice. Fairness and the equal distribution of benefits and burdens.

Adapted from Johnstone 2004

Which is more important, ethics or law?

This is a complicated question with no clear-cut answer. Law and ethics are not the same, but often overlap. Law describes the minimum standards of acceptable behaviour. Ethics describes the highest moral codes of behaviour.

What is an ethical dilemma?

A dilemma is defined as a problem where there is a choice to be made between options that seem equally unfavourable. A moral or ethical dilemma is even more complex. There may be conflicting moral principles that apply equally in a given situation and neither can be chosen without violating the other.

Consider the case of a nurse who accepts the moral principle that demands sanctity of life, but who also accepts the moral principle of non-maleficence, which demands that people should be spared intolerable suffering. Imagine this nurse caring for a person who is terminally ill and suffering intolerable and intractable pain. In this situation, if the nurse accepts the sanctity-of-life principle, he or she would not be able to sanction the administration of the large and potentially lethal doses of narcotics that may be required to alleviate the patient's pain. On the other hand, if the principle of non-maleficence were followed, the nurse might be required to administer potentially lethal dose of narcotics, even though this would probably hasten the patient's death.

In this situation the nurse is confronted with a profound dilemma. To uphold the sanctity-of-life principle would violate the principle of non-maleficence, and to uphold the principle of non-maleficence might violate the sanctity-of-life principle. In everyday nursing practice, the nurse would be guided by both principles; however, the ultimate question for the nurse in this situation is 'Which ethical principle should I choose?'

Johnstone 2004, p 51

In another case, a nurse was caring for a patient from a traditional Greek background who had been diagnosed with metastatic cancer. The doctor had ordered that the patient not be told his diagnosis. However, the patient kept asking the nurse and his family for information about his condition. The family knew the diagnosis, but wanted the doctor to tell the patient. The nurse was caught between a duty to tell the patient the truth as he was requesting (to promote the patient's right to autonomy), and a duty to respect the family's wishes. The nurse was also bound by the requirement to follow the doctor's orders.

The question for the nurse in this situation is, again, 'Which duty ought I to follow: my duty to the patient, to his family or the doctor?'

Johnstone 2004, pp 102–103

Ethics is a concept that you will undoubtedly study in your nursing program. You would be wise to consider and reflect upon ethical situations as they arise in your nursing practice, being guided by ethical principles and the Code of Ethics for Nurses in Australia (ANMC 2002). Ethical dilemmas, when they arise, may cause a great deal of distress and emotional turmoil. In these situations, however, you are not alone and by communicating with your colleagues, clinical educator and/or mentor you will often find the support and guidance you need.

Code of Ethics for Nurses in Australia (2002)

This code of ethics outlines the nursing profession's intention to accept the rights of individuals and to uphold these rights in practice. It is complementary to the International Council of Nurses (ICN) Code of Ethics for Nurses (2000). The purpose of this code of ethics is to:

- identify the fundamental moral commitments of the profession.
- provide nurses with a basis for professional and self-reflection on ethical conduct.
- act as a guide to ethical practice.
- indicate to the community the moral values that nurses can be expected to hold.

Tips and tales 4.6
Crossing over the line

As a nursing student you will have many roles apart from that of a health professional. These roles may include neighbour, family member, friend and community member, among others. There may be times when the boundaries between your roles seem to blur. An example of this is when you become aware that one of the patients on your ward is someone you know. There are specific 'boundaries of practice' guidelines to help you when this type of situation occurs. The following section is adapted from the New South Wales Nurses and Midwives Board Boundaries of Practice document (Nurses Registration Board New South Wales 1999).

What are 'boundaries'?

Boundaries are limits to appropriate behaviour in our personal and professional relationships. In Australia, phrases such as 'crossing over the line' and 'overstepping the mark' are commonly used to describe inappropriate behaviour. Professional boundaries in nursing are defined as limits that protect the space between the professional's power and the patient's vulnerability (Petersen 1992).

What purpose do boundaries serve?

Maintaining appropriate boundaries in a nurse–patient relationship facilitates therapeutic practice and results in safe and effective care. On the one hand, nurses and nursing students may be too cold, distant or formal, so as to not be caring enough to be helpful, and, on the other hand, they may be overly involved, too interested, 'touchy-feely' or invasive. The creation of even a platonic relationship with a patient during a therapeutic relationship increases patient vulnerability, as does caring for a patient that you know from work, university or your community. There is a need to ensure that the nurse–patient relationship is always conducted with the sole intent of benefiting the patient. Knowing the difference between a professional and a personal relationship and being able to recognise boundaries between them may seem like common sense. However, recognition of these boundaries requires knowledge and skills that are acquired through time and experience. Consider the following situation.

A student nurse (James) was undertaking a clinical placement in a mental health unit when a fellow student (Jenny) was admitted following her attempted suicide. James did not know Jenny well but decided to call in and say hello to her. During the course of the next week James spent a lot of time with Jenny, believing his support to be therapeutic. Jenny opened up to him, sharing many details about her life. James began to disclose his own experiences of depression and how it was managed.

On return to university James happened to mention to some fellow students 'in confidence' that Jenny had been admitted to the mental health unit where he undertook his clinical placement. He hoped that they would be sensitive to the situation and understanding when Jenny returned to university. As often happens 'news' spread and Jenny found out. She was devastated that James had broken her trust, even more so because she had shared so many sensitive details about her life with him. Jenny decided not to return to university. James was reported for misconduct.

Consider the implications of the above situation. The outcome could have been avoided if James had recognised and understood the professional boundaries of practice. As a student you may not have enough experience to guide your decisions. We suggest that you consult someone who has more experience.

Coaching tips

- Inform your educator, mentor or nurse unit manager immediately if you become aware of the presence of someone you know when on a clinical placement.
- Refer to education and healthcare policies. Policy directives may mean that you are not to have direct responsibility for the care of a patient you know, or you may be requested to complete your clinical placement in an alternative clinical area.
- Keep interactions with patients you know to a minimum.
- Remember always to maintain complete confidentiality regarding the admission and care of all patients, including people you know.
- Review Chapter 1, where confidentiality is covered in more detail.

Tips and tales 4.7
Punctuality and reliability

Punctuality and reliability are concepts often discussed in relation to work ethic. We need to consider what our ethics (or moral principles) are in regards to work, how these will be judged as good or bad, or right or wrong, and how they affect others.

Consider the following story. While it does not specifically focus on the student's role, the principles are nevertheless crucial to your understanding of professionalism.

Jeremy was a student nurse who had been employed as an assistant in nursing in operating theatres. At 7.15 a.m. after a long, tiring night shift, Jeremy was looking forward to having a rest. The night had seen multiple trauma cases come through into the emergency operating theatre unit. He had just received word that an accident had occurred in a nearby factory and several 'urgent' patients were on their way to the theatre. The day-shift staff would soon be on duty to care for these patients. Unfortunately, the nurse replacing Jeremy had slept in. This meant that Jeremy was required to stay back and work beyond his allocated shift, which had the potential to compromise patient and staff safety, as Jeremy was tired.

The consequences of the nurse's sleep-in are several:

- Urgent care required by the patient is undertaken by tired night staff. A nurse is less able to concentrate after a long, busy shift.
- The changeover of staff when the new shift member arrives will require the 'scrubbing in' of another person, giving rise to potential risks when standards of care are interrupted.
- Staff relationships may be compromised when they are called upon to work longer hours. This could contribute to a reduction of tolerance in the work environment.

Coaching tips

- A good work ethic means that you are punctual for all shifts, meetings and appointments.
- Reflect upon your own practices and identify barriers that prevent you from being punctual.
- Be organised and prepare your uniform and clinical placement requirements in advance.
- Notify the appropriate person/s if an untoward event occurs that prevents you from being on time.
- For new placements, trial and time the trip to the placement location (at the same time of the day, if possible).
- Allow plenty of time to get to the ward or unit, as there may be some distance to walk from the car park or public transport stop.

Tips and tales 4.8
Taking the initiative

Something to think about...

As defined by the *Concise Macquarie Dictionary*, to initiate is to begin, to set something going, and to take the initiative is to take the step or to lead into action.

Clinical experience is an integral and valuable component of student learning (Clare et al 2003). While clinical educators, clinicians, and patient care requirements provide opportunities for students to develop clinical competence and to link theory with practice, students themselves must take the initiative to grow and learn during their clinical placement.

Taking the initiative can be demonstrated in many actions, and students who show initiative are well regarded by team members. This leads to a positive relationship between students and clinicians, in turn assisting student learning and contributing to increased confidence (Clare et al 2003).

Clinical educators and mentors expect students to achieve their learning objectives during their placement experiences. Inherent in this expectation is that students be self-directed and actively contribute to their own needs, making choices and decisions about learning (Reilly & Oermann 1992). Responsibility for learning therefore rests with students.

The following story shows how one student took the initiative.

Jaimie always arrived early for clinical placements. When she arrived on this particular day, the clinicians were resuscitating a patient. Although Jaimie wasn't scheduled to start her shift at this time, she suggested to the clinicians that she could assist by getting patients ready for breakfast, showering them and completing their observations. Jaimie's action supported the clinicians while they were caring for a critical patient. Later they thanked Jaimie for her initiative. Her contribution to the nursing team had ensured all patients received full care.

Jaimie's story shows how initiative can result in a positive outcome. However, students don't always display initiative, as demonstrated by the following story.

Leo, a first-year nursing student, was allocated to a busy medical ward. On the second day of his placement, his clinical educator approached him about some of the problems that had been identified with his practice. Some of the issues were: Leo spent much of his time at the nurses' station rather than with his patients; he was missing from the ward on several occasions; and he had not showered his allocated patients or made their beds.

Was Leo lacking in initiative? What may be the underlying issues for Leo? The discussion between Leo and his clinical educator highlights several perspectives. Leo said he was not confident in undertaking patient care. He admitted he had not attended all classes that semester and had not practised his skills before his placement. He was afraid to ask for help because he thought staff would see him as 'hopeless' and he did not want to fail his clinical placement. He did not feel comfortable and that is why he left the ward when he was asked to provide personal care to patients.

The clinical staff were concerned because he was not reliable and did not undertake nursing care as requested.

Coaching tips

- Be self-directed and ensure that you are thoroughly prepared for clinical placements.
- Seek out opportunities for learning by communicating well thought-out clinical objectives that marry theoretical learning with potential clinical opportunities.
- Be proactive in organising your own clinical learning opportunities.
- Attend inservice sessions when available.

Tips and tales 4.9
Putting work ahead of your studies

Clashes between work, study, clinical placements and personal commitments often cause problems for nursing students. Competing commitments can have an impact on your progress and achieving your goals. Thoughtful, advanced planning can prevent later problems. Be mindful that the effects of celebrations, fatigue, travel, illness, alcohol and drugs may lead you to be unproductive on placement rather than motivated and committed to learn. Consider Kait's story.

Kait was in her third and final year of the nursing program and was also working at her local hospital as an assistant in nursing (undergraduate student). She worked Friday, Saturday and Sunday nights routinely and sometimes picked up other shifts during holiday periods. Kait felt pressured at times to undertake additional shifts. She wanted to be seen as interested, motivated and hard working and was keen to secure a position there as a registered nurse after her graduation. She did not discuss her roster with her manager, even though Kait knew that she would be undertaking a full-time clinical placement in her final semester. She continued to work her routine hours and added additional shifts when requested.

During Kait's clinical placement, the mentor informed her lecturer that Kait was performing adequately, but because Kait's apparent tiredness was of concern it had been decided not to ask her to care for any complex patients, or to undertake any advanced skills. She was not permitted to administer medication and was allocated showering, feeding and bed-making only. Staff felt that it was not safe for Kait to perform care commensurate with her educational level.

Further discussions between the mentor and the lecturer revealed that Kait had already been sent home on the previous day because she was tired. When she had admitted that she had worked the previous night shift, she had been sent home for safety reasons.

In the above scenario, what issues can be identified?

- Patient safety is the most important issue that needs to be considered. Kait has a responsibility to undertake care to the level of her knowledge in a safe, accountable manner. Her tiredness detracted from her ability to perform safely.

- Kait was required to undertake compulsory clinical placement as a component of her studies, meeting learning goals and undertaking patient care. She was unable to achieve this outcome during her placement experience.

- Educational institutions have in place policies that guide student behaviour, both in the classroom and on clinical placements. At Kait's institution, her behaviour contravened those policies, and this then resulted in a case of misconduct.

It is important to maintain a 'life in balance'—this includes your psychological, physical, social, spiritual and environmental health. Allow time for study and make thoughtful decisions about where your energy is to be spent. You must be at 'full capacity' on clinical placement to ensure that you provide safe nursing care and can learn effectively.

Coaching tips

- Be accountable, safe and responsible for all practice undertaken.
- Plan all activities in advance and avoid clashes between work, other commitments and clinical learning experiences.
- Prioritise and organise your life.

Tips and tales 4.10
Getting the support you need

There may be times during your clinical placements when you need support in some way or another. Support services are available at your educational institution during your placements, but it may require extra effort to access these services (due to your placement shifts). The healthcare facility also has many support services and some of these may be available to you, dependent on your requirements and the service's access criteria. If you are accessing support through healthcare facilities, you may have to pay for some services.

When you are involved in the care of others, you may sometimes feel compelled to talk about your own issues. If a problem has the potential to affect safe practice, your clinical educator or mentor may be required to take action and to inform the appropriate body at your university or college.

Table 4.1 lists some of the support mechanisms that may be available to you before, during and after your clinical placement. Of course available support may vary according to the nature of your placement, the educational institution that you are enrolled in, and the study mode that you are undertaking. Be proactive in identifying support mechanisms early in your student life. It is easier to access and use the services if you know about them in advance, rather than to start from scratch when you have a problem.

Table 4.1 Where to find support during clinical placement

Type of support	Services available
Academic	• Learning workshops associated with mathematics and drug calculations • Writing assistance (e.g. for nursing report writing) • Peer mentoring (e.g. for nursing skill development or feedback on skill performance) • Web-based programs: identification of learning styles (see also <www.metamath.com/multiple/multiple_choice_questions.html> or <www.engr.ncsu.edu/learningstyles/ilsweb.html>)
Counselling services	• Personal development (e.g. how to get along with difficult people, or how to gain insight into your behaviour) • Discussion of clinical issues (e.g. caring for a person who is dying) • Stress-management strategies • Time-management strategies

Continued

Table 4.1 Where to find support during clinical placement *(continued)*

Type of support	Services available
Chaplains	Discussion of experiences and feelings from clinical or pastoral care
Special needs assistance	Welfare support to attend clinical placements, financial or student loans, crisis care, child support etc
Accommodation	Available through some healthcare institutions (ask your clinical coordinator or check the institution's website)
Language (students from non-English-speaking background)	Advice available from • The international unit at their educational institution • The academic support unit
Scholarships	*Healthcare institution scholarships* • Helping-hand (to purchase the uniform) • International exchange to experience a placement overseas • Fee support *Workplace scholarships* Study leave, fee support for a clinical placement *State or territory health department* Undergraduate nursing scholarship or assistance to attend special placements (e.g. rural placements) For details see websites of your healthcare institution, state/territory government, registration board, professional groups and associations
Advocacy	• Clinical educators • Mentors • Lecturers or other staff at the educational institution • Clinical coordinator (education- or facility-based) • Student bodies or associations • Professional organisations (e.g. nursing colleges)

Continued

Table 4.1 Where to find support during clinical placement *(continued)*

Type of support	Services available
Policy breach assistance (e.g. harassment, bullying, privacy issues)	As for advocacy
General practitioners, emergency departments	• Medical assistance associated with clinical placement: • Immunisations before entry into a health facility • Advice about medical problems before a placement • Medical clearance before a placement • Treatment for a needlestick injury • Other injury during placement
Disability advisors	• How particular disabilities can affect you on placement • Resources and avenues for assistance that may be available Registration for this service is required in most educational institutions; placements are dependent on your ability to provide safe nursing care

Activity

Investigate the student support services that are available at your educational and healthcare institutions. Identify how these services can be of support to you during clinical placement.

Reflective thinking activities

Self-assessment

Complete this self-assessment to help you understand who you are and what is important to you as a nurse.

What types of clinical placement have I most preferred? Why?

(e.g. I preferred placements that were not fast-paced. I had time to sit and talk to my patients and I felt I could ask lots of questions because the staff were not rushed.)

What types of clinical placement have I least preferred? Why?

(e.g. I sometimes felt overwhelmed in the fast-paced, highly technical placements, and did not always feel I could contribute.)

What motivates and inspires me to be the best nurse I can be?

(e.g. Good role models who are skilled, knowledgable and excited to be nurses; positive feedback from other nurses and patients.)

What is most important to me when I am nursing?

(e.g. Learning something new every day; knowing I've made a difference in one person's life; feeling part of the nursing team.)

I made a difference on a clinical placement when…

(e.g. I was able to advocate for a patient who was in a lot of pain, so that a different type of analgesia was ordered for him.)

My greatest strengths as a nurse are…

(e.g. Eagerness and motivation; communication skills with staff and patients.)

My limitations as a nurse are…

(e.g. Not enough confidence to challenge nursing care that is not best practice; documentation; patient assessment skills.)

Reality check

What type of feedback have I received from patients, nursing staff and my educators about my strengths?

What type of feedback have I received from patients, nursing staff and my educators about my limitations?

_____

_____

_____

How did my self-assessment compare with others' assessment of me?

_____

_____

_____

What will I do to enhance my strengths and address my limitations? (Be very realistic and strategic.)

_____

_____

_____

Whose support and guidance do I need to help me enhance my strengths and address my limitations?

_____

_____

_____

References

ANMC 2002 Code of ethics for nurses in Australia. Australian Nursing and Midwifery Council. Online. Available <www.anmc.org.au>, 1 April 2006.

Baly M (ed) 1991 As Miss Nightingale said. Scutari Press, London.

Boud D 1999 Avoiding the traps: seeking good practice in the use of self-assessment and reflection in professional courses. Social Work Education 18(2):121–132.

Bourgeois S 2006 An archive of caring for nursing. PhD thesis, University of Western Sydney, Penrith.

Buresh B & Gordon S 2000 From silence to voice. What nurses know and must communicate to the public. Cornell University Press, New York.

Chenevert M 1985 Pro-nurse handbook. Designed for the nurse who wants to thrive professionally. Mosby, St Louis.

Clare J, Brown D, Edwards H et al 2003 Evaluating clinical learning environments: creating education-practice partnerships and clinical education benchmarks for nursing. Learning outcomes and curriculum development in major disciplines: Nursing phase 2 final report. School of Nursing & Midwifery, Flinders University, Adelaide.

Crow GL 2000 Knowing self. In FL Bower (ed), Nurses taking the lead: personal qualities of effective leadership, pp 15–37. WB Saunders, Philadelphia.

Dahnke M & Dreher M 2006 Defining ethics and applying theories. In V Lachman (ed), Applied ethics in nursing. Springer, New York.

Driscoll J 2000 Practising clinical supervision. A reflective approach. Ballière Tindall, Edinburgh.

International Council of Nurses 2000 Code of ethics for nurses. International Council of Nurses, Geneva.

Johnstone M 2004 Bioethics: a nursing perspective, 4th edn. Churchill Livingstone, Sydney.

Leininger MM 1991 The theory of culture care diversality and universality. In MM Leininger (ed), Culture care diversity & universality: a theory of nursing, pp 5–68. National League for Nursing, New York.

Nurses Registration Board New South Wales 1999 A project report to the Nurses Registration Board of New South Wales on the development of guidelines for registered nurses and enrolled nurses regarding the boundaries of practice. Online. Available <www.nursesreg.nsw.gov.au/bounds/report.htm>, 16 April 2004.

Orem D 1991 Nursing concepts of practice, 3rd edn. McGraw-Hill, New York.

Petersen M 1992 At personal risk: boundary violations in professional–client relationships. WW Norton, New York.

Reilly DE & Oermann MH 1992 Clinical teaching in nursing education. National League for Nursing, New York.

van Manen M 1990 Researching lived experience. State University of New York Press, New York.

Walsh M & Walsh A 1999 Measuring patient satisfaction with nursing care: experience using the Newcastle satisfaction with nursing scale. Journal of Advanced Nursing 29(2):307–315.

Watson J 1999 Postmodern nursing and beyond. Churchill Livingstone, Edinburgh.

Watson R, Stimpson A, Topping A et al 2002 Clinical competence assessment in nursing: a systematic review of the literature. Journal of Advanced Nursing 39(5):421–431.

Williams AM 1998 The delivery of quality nursing care: a grounded theory study of the nurse's perspective. Journal of Advanced Nursing 27:808–816.

Chapter 5

How you communicate

Envision how things would be if the voice and visibility of nursing were commensurate with the size and importance of nursing in health care.

Buresh & Gordon 2000, p 11

Tips and tales 5.1
What is a nurse?

In this section we draw from the work of Bernice Buresh and Suzanne Gordon, two journalists who have written extensively on the importance of nurses being able to define and promote their profession.

The public holds nurses in very high regard. Opinion polls indicate that nurses are the most highly rated profession in terms of honesty and ethics, rating significantly higher than pharmacists, teachers or doctors. Yet studies indicate that when people think of registered nurses they are more inclined to dwell on their kindness and caring than on their knowledge, expertise or professionalism. The public's awareness of nurses' professionalism is linked to nurses' ability to highlight their experience, skills and expertise.

> The job at hand for nurses is to help the public (as well as other health care professionals) to construct an authentic meaning of the word 'nurse' that conveys the richness and uniqueness of nursing. This means not misconstruing nursing as something commonplace, but deepening the public's comprehension of nursing as deeply complex, skilled and essential to patient care. (Buresh & Gordon 2000, p 17)

Coaching tips

How do you introduce yourself?

Nurses have a choice about the way they present themselves to patients, families, doctors, other clinicians and the general public. They can present themselves in ways that assert their personal and professional identity, or they can remain part of the wider, undifferentiated healthcare services industry. They can highlight their clinical knowledge and competence, or they can conceal it. Each day in the workplace, what nurses say and do can elicit the respect and collegial treatment their professional standing deserves, or undermine it. While caring for patients and families, or interacting with other members of the healthcare team, nurses convey messages about their own respect for the status of nursing. Some of these messages are implicit; others are more explicit, delivered through presentation, body language, tone of voice and conversational style.

Some examples to think about...

If a nurse thinks it advisable to consult a doctor, she or he can inform the patient by saying, 'I'll discuss this with the doctor'. By using these words nurses imply that they have clinical knowledge and judgment, and see themselves as doctors' colleagues. Alternatively nurses can act in a subservient way by saying, 'I'll have to ask the doctor'.

When contacting a doctor, a nurse can establish collegiality by beginning the conversation with the words 'Hello Dr Smith, this is Sarah O'Shea (or Nurse O'Shea), Mrs Johnson's nurse. She is experiencing chest pain and I think...'. Alternatively, she can cast herself in an inferior role by beginning 'I'm so sorry to bother you Dr Smith, but this is Sarah, Mrs Johnson's nurse...'.

The way that nurses introduce themselves to patients and their families can also have a significant impact on how they are perceived. You can introduce yourself with a firm handshake, provide your full name, inform them that you are a student nurse and explain your role in the patient's care. Or you can simply say, 'Hello, I'm John' and leave it at that.

Most patients meeting you for the first time have few visual cues about your identity and role. Your introduction is your best opportunity to let people know that you are a student nurse, a serious professional with clinical skills and knowledge. Being serious and professional is not the same as being distant and aloof. It simply means presenting yourself as a knowledgable caregiver. This presentation tends to reassure patients rather than alienate them.

First name basis?

In Australia it has become increasingly common for nurses to use only their first names when introducing themselves to patients, visitors or doctors. Even some name badges bear only first names. Although society has become more informal, can you imagine doctors introducing themselves by their first names only? Why then is there an imbalance between these two professions? If nurses continue to uphold and reinforce these identification practices, it suggests that nurses regard doctors as superior in the healthcare environment. We know that this is not the real intention of nurses who use only their first names. Mostly they are doing it to develop a friendly and informal relationship with their patients, and to show them that they are 'on their side' or 'an equal'. Unfortunately, this often misconstrues what patients really want and need from a nurse. They don't want a friend; they want a nurse with knowledge and skill. 'A really good nurse will establish the context for a relationship. They will communicate to a patient: This is what I do. This is what you do. This is what I know. I will make sure that everything will be all right for you' (Buresh & Gordon 2000, p 52).

Tips and tales 5.2
Welcome to Australia

This section is related to the topic of cultural competence discussed in Chapter 3. It is written especially for international students, although it will undoubtedly be of benefit to local students who want to better understand and support their peers. We hope that this brief overview will complement what you learn in class about contemporary practice cultures in Australia and help you to become accustomed to the clinical learning environment and the diverse factors that affect your learning experience. Without this knowledge, miscommunication is common and learning possibilities sometimes reduced.

Firstly and most importantly, we'd like to say welcome to Australia. The increasing numbers of international students in academic programs such as nursing have had a positive impact on our ability to appreciate and understand different cultures. The diversity and richness you bring to the academic and clinical environment enhances the learning opportunities of all students and staff.

While most students will at some stage experience difficulties related to their clinical placement, these may be exacerbated by language and cultural differences. If you experience problems, it is important to reflect upon, try to distinguish and analyse the root cause of the problems so that appropriate support, guidance and teaching can be provided. Try to identify your fundamental issues of concern from the coaching tips below (adapted from Remedios & Webb 2005).

Coaching tips

Receptive communication (verbal and non-verbal)

Do you sometimes find it hard to understand what your patients or nursing colleagues are saying to you? Local accents, shortened, fast speech and the use of colloquialisms may cause significant difficulties for international students. Misunderstandings between you and others may occur if you do not readily acknowledge when you have not understood or have only partially understood a conversation. Most importantly, patients' safety may be jeopardised if you are not perfectly clear about what is being asked of you. Initially it may be culturally difficult for you to do this, but keep in mind that in Australia it is not considered disrespectful to question an individual in authority or to ask someone to repeat what they have said. Nor is it considered a 'failure' on your part if you have not understood something. On the contrary, clinicians will expect you to ask questions, and to ask for clarification whenever you need to.

Strategies for improvement

- If you want to confirm your understanding of an instruction or discussion, try paraphrasing: for example, 'Can I confirm that you'd like me to take Mrs Smith to the shower on a commode, because of her low blood pressure?'
- Ask others to explain any colloquial language you do not understand.
- If you are unsure of healthcare terminology related to the patient mix on the ward where you are undertaking your placement, ask questions and be prepared to do some research.
- Remember, nodding or silence following a conversation may be taken to indicate that you fully understood what was being said, even if the reverse is true.

Expressive communication (verbal and non-verbal)

Do you sometimes find it difficult and frustrating trying to make yourself understood by patients or nursing colleagues? In Australia you'll be expected to be fluent in the English language, familiar with colloquialisms and conversant with the professional language used for reporting and communicating with health professionals, but still have the ability to switch to less formal language when needed—for example, when conversing with patients.

Strategies for improvement

- Observing nursing staff communicating effectively with one another and with patients will allow you to compare this with what you are used to, help you clarify expectations and enable you to build upon what you already know.
- Reflect on these observations carefully. Ask yourself what made the interactions effective. How and why was humour used? What colloquialisms and terms need clarification?
- Make the most of opportunities to practise communicating with patients and staff.

- Do not hesitate to ask your clinical educator or mentor to observe you and provide detailed feedback on your progress.
- Most educational institutions have student support services that provide English language tuition. Avail yourself of this opportunity if you require additional help.

Written communication

Is it difficult to understand what is written or to find the English words for what you want to write? Both international and local students can experience difficulties with reading and writing. Patients' notes, referral letters, medication charts and other forms of professional documentation may be especially problematic as students try to find and use appropriate language and grammar.

Strategies for improvement

- Practise, practise, practise! Try writing a nursing report on note-paper and asking someone you respect and trust to critique it for you before you write in a patient's notes.
- Reading nursing journals will help you to develop your fluency in English and your professional vocabulary, and will build on what you already know.
- Even reading good quality English-language novels set in Australia will improve your literacy and grammar, and help you to better understand colloquialisms and local culture. Ask your librarian to recommend appropriate novels.
- Remember that in nursing reports you must always sign your name in English.

Cultural issues

Are you finding the clinical culture in Australia confusing and stressful? If you have no previous experience with Western healthcare systems, it will be difficult at first to understand the complexity of the structures and values operating within the system. The interactions between you and patients or fellow students may present unique problems. This not only applies to international students but also to local students caring for patients from diverse cultures. Misunderstandings may involve religion, gender and age-related issues, as well as language. Sometimes the lack of understanding and tolerance on the part of clinical staff and fellow students may have a negative impact on the ability of international students to fit into and feel accepted in the clinical environment.

Strategies for improving understanding

- Many educational institutions have dedicated courses or at least an orientation program to prepare students for the cultural differences they may encounter. Local community colleges also provide programs to assist with reading, writing and speaking. Make the most of these learning opportunities as well as the opportunities to interact with local students.
- Join local sporting, musical or recreational clubs to increase your opportunities for socialising with people from different backgrounds.
- During your clinical placement experience it is important that you express any concerns you have, even though it may be difficult to do so. Sharing your worries with someone you trust will mean that you can be supported and guided. Sadly, not all students, staff or patients will be sensitive to different health beliefs, customs, and cultural and religious practices. If you experience discrimination, subtle or obvious, you need to discuss it with your educator or academic staff member. All Australian educational and healthcare institutions have policies regarding discrimination and your concerns will be taken seriously.
- Seek out a peer mentor to work with during your studies. This should be a person who can support your development in the English language. Spend time together focusing on language development and understanding.

- *Everyday English for nursing* (Grice 2003) is an excellent resource to help you develop your English language skills.

Tips and tales 5.3
Using professional language

Nurses must be able to describe the care they give and the clinical decisions they make (Buresh & Gordon 2000). In discussions with colleagues, patients, their significant others and the public, the language that nurses use reflects on their professional standing. Nursing students are recognised as a part of this group of professionals and are expected to behave according to the conventions of the nursing profession.

You will accumulate professional and jargon-based words and statements that will become a normal part of your practice language. Nursing jargon refers to words that are used by nurses when they talk about their practice. These words may exclude people who are unfamiliar with their use, so choose your words carefully when you speak to people who do not have a nursing background. Distinguish between what you say to health workers and what you say to the lay person (Buresh & Gordon 2000). Colloquial language, or slang, is often referred to as conversational speech without constraint. While appropriate perhaps in some contexts, its use should be minimised in the practice environment.

For some nurses, it is not unusual for them to address their patients, particularly if they are elderly, using an endearment (sweetie, cherub, darling, dahls, angel, lovey etc) (Gardner & Johnson 2001). However, many patients will be offended by being addressed in this manner, so don't assume that it is acceptable. A good rule is to simply ask a patient if he would prefer you to use his given name (e.g. John) or address him more formally (Mr Smith).

As you progress through your nursing program, you will develop a wide repertoire of professional terminology. Give careful consideration to your audience to ensure that you use the most appropriate language in each situation. Nursing terminology and medical terms are words that should not be confused. Their inappropriate use will completely change the meaning of your message. Abbreviations must be approved by the institution in which you are undertaking your placement. Some words that are commonly abbreviated can have very different meanings within various contexts of practice.

Coaching tips

- Reflect upon language used in professional situations and how it affects others.
- Take stock of the language you use: words, selected statements (informal and formal), tone and loudness.
- Consider who you are speaking to and their age, culture, medical condition, status and knowledge.
- Consider the words, statements and conventions of language that are appropriate in each situation.
- Select words that cannot easily be misinterpreted.
- Explain medical and nursing terms to patients using language that is easily understood.
- Be aware that a word may have several meanings.
- Be aware that the way a word is interpreted may be influenced by thoughts, feelings and beliefs people may have about that word (e.g. drug versus medication, or miscarriage versus abortion).
- Avoid the use of colloquial and coarse language in the practice environment (many people are offended by swearing).
- Consider the effect of words on others (some words may convey a false sense of urgency to a patient).
- Learn the meaning of medical terminology and use the terms accurately (e.g. words ending in -ectomy, -ology, -oscopy, -otomy etc).

- Make a list of accepted abbreviations.
- Listen to the way your role model uses professional language.
- Consider that the use of certain words may offend, alienate, or detract from your intended meaning.

Tips and tales 5.4
Patient handover

The patient handover report is a communication practice used by nurses and other allied health carers to communicate nursing care requirements, patients' conditions and progress at change of shift. Crisp and Taylor state that 'The purpose of the [handover] report is to provide continuity of care amongst nurses who are caring for a patient' (2005, p 483). These reports may be given verbally in person, taped or written.

In some institutions handovers may be undertaken as patient rounds, with patients and their families also contributing to decision-making and care-planning. In others, handovers may be held in the staff room or conference room, with nurses from the previous shift joined by nurses for the next shift. In these situations the handover time is an opportunity for nurses to come together to discuss patient care as a team. Because of time constraints reports are sometimes taped. The advantage of taping is that nurses can provide their handover at a convenient time during the shift, but this doesn't allow nurses to clarify and review care as they would in a face-to-face handover.

Change-of-shift reports should be conducted efficiently to enable one group to leave and the other group to begin the shift. The handover report describes the health status of patients, any aberrations from normal, interventions implemented and the effectiveness of interventions (such as analgesia). Information needs to be accurate, objective, concise, logical and to the point.

It is important for students to make the most of opportunities to be present at patient handover reports. Practise giving and receiving handover about your patient's condition and care requirements. Ask your mentor for advice and feedback about your handover.

Coaching tips

- Be on time for shift handover and remain for the entire process.
- Take notes and ask questions about anything you are unsure of.
- Be respectful of the people you are discussing. Avoid the use of judgmental language, and do not label or stereotype your patients or make negative comments about them.
- Use correct terminology, professional language and only easily understood and recognised abbreviations.
- Avoid repetition and irrelevant data.
- Discuss with your clinical educator or mentor issues that need clarification.

Tips and tales 5.5
Your voice in the clinical environment

Your voice is one of your most effective communication tools. You should be aware how you use this tool, and make it an efficient mechanism in your repertoire of skills. Reflect upon the pitch and tone of your voice so that you are aware of how you come across to others. The following are some extreme examples:

- a nurse calling down the corridor
- speaking so quietly that your patients cannot hear what you are saying
- a group of nurses laughing loudly at the nurses' station

Clinical environments are different in structure and design. They can be small, intimate rooms where patients are interviewed, or rooms attached to a long corridor. Corridors echo and the sound of people's voices can carry over long distances and traverse hard surfaces such as doors and walls. A comment made to a patient in one room may be very appropriate, but if the comment is overheard in an adjoining room it may unnecessarily frighten or distress someone. Think carefully about the pitch of your voice when talking to others.

Pitch of voice is critical to the development of appropriate communication skills. A loud voice is easily heard, but also easily overheard. Some people find that their voice projects well and other people have no trouble hearing what they say. People with this type of voice need to be mindful of how far their voice carries. If you are aware that you have a loud voice, try standing next to the person you are talking to rather than speaking from a distance. This technique has the effect of reducing the projection factor you add to your voice when speaking at a distance (even short distances). Use eye contact to help direct your voice.

On the other hand, a soft voice can be difficult to hear and detracts from the message being conveyed. It can be a source of frustration for the listener. If you have a very soft voice, remember that any physical barriers (such as masks, or curtains around a bed) may render your voice difficult to hear. Keep what you say clear, simple and straightforward. Connect with those to whom you are speaking to engage their attention (maintain eye contact, position yourself, use appropriate gestures). Practice voice projection to enable your voice to be heard within a group. Move forward in a group to engage people in the conversation so that you are speaking within a closer range.

Accents have a powerful effect on the listener's ability to understand what is being said. If you speak with an accent, you may need to slow your speech to allow the listener to 'attune' to the accent initially so that communication is effective.

Coaching tips

- Assess your voice—is it too loud or too soft for effective communication? Try taping yourself and then listening to the tape. Ask family or friends to give you some feedback about how you sound.

- Walk up to people to communicate rather than using a broadcast format.
- Consider the number of people that need to hear you and the type of information that it is important to convey. Reflect upon the situation and modify your voice to suit.
- Be aware of how you sound during spoken communication practices. Is your voice squeaky, high-pitched, growling or guttural?
- Consider how fast or slowly you speak, and the associated pitch of your voice.
- Be careful of how your voice projects in long corridors or large rooms.
- If you are concerned about your voice and the impact it has on others, seek feedback, and try to improve your speech by attending training sessions or public speaking groups.

Tips and tales 5.6
Telephones and the internet

The use of telephones and the internet as communication tools in modern society has progressed rapidly. While both forms of communication are certainly convenient they can also be intrusive and annoying. Because telephones and the internet are essential for workplace communication, there are some guidelines that you should be aware of.

Clinical facilities have policies that govern the use of telephones and the internet. Ward or unit telephones and computers are the property of the healthcare institution and financial costs are associated with their use. Unless it is essential for you to make a personal phone call or to send an urgent email, remember that the telephones and computers are for business use only. Using a telephone for personal calls may prevent other healthcare staff from using it to give or receive information relevant to patient care.

Similarly, spending time on the ward computer prevents others from using it for more important patient-care purposes.

When you start on each new ward, ask what the policies are regarding telephone and internet access. In some facilities students are not to answer telephones or to give out patient information, and in many situations internet access is restricted to staff only.

Telephone etiquette

When you use the telephone you'll be expected to use appropriate telephone etiquette.

- Answer the telephone promptly.
- Begin the conversation with your name, designation and location.
- Discontinue any conversation or activity before answering the telephone (such as eating, typing etc).
- Speak clearly and distinctly, using a pleasant tone of voice.
- Inform the caller when you are putting them on 'hold', and press the 'hold' button, so they do not overhear other conversations that may be held at the nursing station.
- Tell callers what your actions will be before you undertake them (e.g. I am going to transfer you to another number).
- Always be courteous, friendly and ready to assist the caller.
- Pass on messages promptly—it is best to write the messages down rather than rely on your memory.

A mobile phone is now far more than just a telephone and is often referred to as a multi-media device with wireless connectivity. In the clinical learning environment a mobile phone has the potential to cause interference with technological equipment and most health institutions request you to turn it off as you enter.

Your use of mobile phones during placement needs to be carefully considered. Making and receiving calls or text messaging should be done only in your breaks, if urgent. You will be expected to leave your mobile phone in your bag or locker and not carry it with you.

You should also take care when using your phone as a multi-media device. Consider the following scenario.

Nikos had been allocated to the special care nursery for his clinical placement. He was very excited and enthusiastic about this placement, as it was an area that he had selected for his graduate year. During the course of his placement, Nikos came across a baby who had a severe birth deformity. To help him to remember the condition, he took a series of photos using his mobile phone, so that he could develop a learning portfolio.

At his debrief session, Nikos shared his learning ideas with the other students and his clinical educator. Nikos had not sought written consent for the photos of the baby, and by using his mobile phone in this way he had unknowingly contravened the educational and healthcare institutions' policies.

Here are some other instances of where phones have been used inappropriately:

- texting messages to friends during the handover report
- listening to music on a mobile phone, wearing earpieces, while carrying out patient care for patients with disabilities
- booking football tickets in the patient's bathroom while the patient was in the next cubicle showering himself
- giving a mobile phone to the patient while changing the patient's dressing, so as not to miss an expected call

Coaching tips

- Develop courteous and effective telephone etiquette. Speak clearly and not too fast.
- Be mindful of the type of information you can divulge over the telephone in your role as a student and to whom.

- Always find out details about the person you are speaking to at the beginning of the call.
- Know the protocols for taking patient care orders, test results and medication prescriptions over the phone and adhere to these conventions strictly.
- Know the healthcare facility's protocols for speaking to the media or the police.
- Always put the principles of confidentiality and privacy into practice when answering telephones during placement.
- When phoning a doctor, be organised. Have the information about the patient ready so you can answer any questions. Make sure you are aware of the patient's clinical condition, recent vital signs and other assessments before you make the call.
- Check for personal phone and text messages only in your breaks.
- Leave your placement location details (ward phone number) with your significant other in case of an emergency.
- Keep the contact details up to date in your student record— telephone and email are often used by lecturers to contact you to clarify learning issues.
- Access the internet only for patient care purposes and with the permission of the appropriate staff.

Telephone order guidelines

- Clarify any telephone orders given by a medical officer.
- Confirm the name of the patient at the beginning of the call.
- Repeat any orders back to the medical officer.
- Where required, a second person should listen to and countersign the order.
- Record the complete order in the patient's notes, including the date and time of the call, and the medical officer's name.

Crisp & Taylor 2005, p 487

Tips and tales 5.7
Self-disclosure

Self-disclosure is an act of revelation. What should you reveal about yourself in the course of your placement and to whom? Should you share your medical history or problems with your clients?

Some clinical placements provide the opportunity for you to attend group meetings. During these meetings, clients often disclose personal information about themselves and at times you may be tempted to share your experiences about a similar problem. Be cautious! The invitation by the group leader to be a part of the group is in your capacity as a nursing student. It is not for you to discuss your personal circumstances, conditions or history. The intention is for you to learn from the global concepts illustrated in the group discussions and to focus on the therapeutic interactions that occur. In group meetings attention should not be drawn away from clients.

The same principles apply if you have the opportunity to be involved in a case conference. Objective, informed discussion that focuses on the clients is the purpose of the meetings. Don't be tempted to disclose personal information about yourself, even if it seems relevant.

While there may be a few instances in which self-disclosure may be appropriate, it should always be well thought-out and never be done to satisfy your own needs (e.g. as a medical consultation or to gain sympathy). Before you engage in self-disclosure, reflect on your own agenda and motivation. Is your self-disclosure a genuine act to help others or a way to satisfy your own needs?

Coaching tips

- Before you join a group counselling session, seek guidelines from the group leader about your role in group meetings.
- Monitor your behaviours to ensure that you do not take attention

away from members of the group (for example, continually swishing your hair, sighing, moving around the room).
- Show respect and listen attentively to members of the group.
- Arrive on time for the group session and wait until the end to leave.
- Avoid talking to fellow students during a group therapy session. The focus is on the patients, and short conversations with a colleague are viewed as disrespectful and can often make patients or other group members angry.
- Do not at any time disclose any personal information. This includes your medical or psychological history (and any other history you may have).
- Save questions until after the meeting—it is not a question and answer session.
- Always thank the group members for allowing you to participate in their session.

Tips and tales 5.8
Providing effective feedback

Feedback is an important component of student learning during clinical placement. It contributes to ongoing improvement when supported by quality feedback mechanisms. Feedback has the power to motivate others and to facilitate change and learning.

The concept of feedback is complex. It provides information about past performance and provides strategies for future learning. The degree to which feedback facilitates change, learning and future performance depends on many factors, including the perception and acceptance of the feedback by the recipient, the way feedback is conveyed, and the personal characteristics of persons involved.

Feedback should not be viewed as a bureaucratic process or a tool for control. It is not about being punitive but offers a mechanism to enhance communication and teamwork. It is a powerful motivator for change. Effective feedback provides the potential to increase self-esteem and workplace satisfaction and is an opportunity to demonstrate that you value others.

Mechanisms for providing feedback may be formal or informal (Penman & Oliver 2004). Formal feedback mechanisms may be hard-copy or online questionnaires that incorporate a rating scale, or forms that request open-ended comments. While you may receive feedback about your clinical performance, you may also be requested to give feedback about your clinical experiences, your mentor or clinical educator. Your feedback needs to be carefully considered, given freely and with the intent to inform and to be honest. For feedback to be most effective, it should be provided immediately following your placement, so that you capture your thoughts, feelings and ideas. You have the right to question whether privacy and confidentiality principles are operational. Informal and spontaneous feedback is also a valuable mechanism to affirm and value others. Do not be afraid to offer constructive feedback during your learning experiences.

Feedback on student performance

You should also expect to receive regular feedback from the nurses you work with and your educator. This may be in the form of a formal evaluation of your clinical performance or as opportunistic feedback that provides you with immediate information about your performance of a specific task or situation.

Feedback needs to be given in an environment conducive to listening and comprehending (quiet and away from the distraction of other people), and at a time when you can pay attention to what is being said. Your willingness to accept and to respond to the feedback is an important factor in the feedback process. Listen attentively, reflect on what is said and be willing to discuss the issues presented. Negotiation and assertiveness skills will allow you to seek and qualify information. Ask for examples to illustrate a particular criterion. Show how you have learnt from situations and moved forward in your learning during the session. Be proactive and ask for strategies that will help you develop further. Your feedback session is not the time to bring up complaints about individuals. Issues of this kind should be dealt with at the time they occur. Most institutions have a mechanism for handling complaints or for commending someone.

Coaching tips

- Take every opportunity to provide feedback and to support quality mechanisms and processes. Remember that your feedback has the power to change practices and is therefore a critical component of your professional life.
- Make constructive comments when providing feedback.
- Mention a positive comment before a negative one.
- Take time to reflect upon your feedback before you submit it.
- Be receptive to feedback about your performance. Actively strive to grow and develop from constructively offered feedback.

Reflective thinking activities

How do you introduce yourself to staff on the first day of a clinical placement?

_____

_____

_____

How do you introduce yourself to your patients when you first meet them?

_____

_____

_____

You are a third-year student. One of the patients you have been caring for is febrile (38.7°C), oxygen saturation level is 89 per cent, and respiratory rate is 34. The registered nurse you are working with is tied up and asks you to phone the doctor. How do you prepare for the phone call and what will you say to the doctor?

_____

_____

_____

Tape yourself giving a simulated patient handover, then critique yourself.

1. What are your impressions of both the content of the handover, the way it was delivered and the way it sounded? Did you focus on the most important aspects of the patient's condition and care? If not, why not?

    _____

    _____

    _____

    _____

2. Did you use the correct terminology? Give examples.

    _____

    _____

    _____

    _____

3. Did you sound confident or timid? How can you improve this?

_____

_____

_____

4. Was your voice clear and articulate or did you mumble and stumble over your words?

_____

_____

_____

5. Were you too loud, too soft or too monotone?

_____

_____

_____

Imagine it is the last day of your clinical placement. You have had some great times there with some wonderful and supportive staff. However, you've also worked with a few registered nurses who made it obvious to you that they resented students. They were dismissive of your questions and unappreciative of your help. Write a letter to the nursing unit manager about your experiences in the unit.

_____

_____

_____

_____

_____

References

Buresh B & Gordon S 2000 From silence to voice. What nurses know and must communicate to the public. Cornell University Press, New York.
Crisp J & Taylor C (eds) 2005 Potter and Perry's fundamentals of nursing, 2nd edn. Mosby, Sydney.

Gardner S & Johnson P 2001 Sexual harassment in healthcare: strategies for employers. Hospital Topics 79(4):5–11.

Grice T 2003 Everyday English for nursing. Elsevier, Edinburgh.

Penman J & Oliver M 2004 Meeting the challenges of assessing clinical placement venues in a Bachelor of Nursing program. Online. Available <http://jutlp.uow.edu.au/2004_v01_i02/penman002.html>, 11 January 2005.

Remedios L & Webb G 2005 Transforming practice through clinical education: professional supervision and mentoring. Elsevier, Sydney.

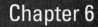

Chapter 6

Insights from clinical experts

Trust one who has gone through it.

Virgil (Roman poet, 70–19 BC), *Aeneid*

Introduction

In this chapter we are delighted to include contributions written by nurses from a wide cross-section of roles and nursing specialties. Each section introduces you to the particular learning opportunities and challenges inherent in these diverse clinical areas. While it has not been possible to cover every clinical specialty, we are sure that the following selection will provide insight into the wonderful opportunities available to nursing students. We are confident that you'll be inspired as these nurses share with you their passion for their work, and motivated as they explain the unique qualities of different practice areas.

This chapter is designed to allow you to prepare for and plan your clinical placements. However, you'll also be able to use it to delve into the different career pathways and specialities that are open to graduates. We hope that you find reading this chapter interesting and thought-provoking.

6.1 Child and adolescent health nursing

Diana Keatinge
Professor, Paediatric, Youth and Family Health
Nursing, University of Newcastle and Hunter
New England Area Health Service

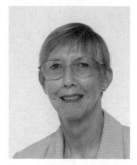

Professor Diana Keatinge

Mosby's Dictionary of medicine, nursing and health professions (2006) identifies childhood as 'the period in human development that extends from birth until the onset of puberty' (p 249), and adolescence as 'the period in development between the onset of puberty and adulthood' (p 45). It is evident from these definitions that child and adolescent health extends from the care of infants right through to young people approximately 18 years old. As many authors note, of central importance when considering child and adolescent health is that healthcare delivery does not take place only for the infant, child or young person as an individual, but rather within the context of his/her family (Harmon Hanson 2005; Wong 1999).

Learning opportunities

Healthcare delivery for infants, children and young people may take place in a community-based facility such as a child and family health clinic, in the home as in the instance of community paediatric nursing or in a hospital environment. The range in age groups encompassed in child and adolescent health, as well as in contexts of service delivery, provides students with learning opportunities in primary and community healthcare delivery, and in acute care. Further, consideration of the child or young person and his or her family as a single unit in the planning and delivery of healthcare, offers the opportunity for students to develop their understanding of factors in society that have an impact on families and the psychosocial and physical health and wellbeing of their members.

Research evidence has determined the importance of a nurturing and stimulating environment in a child's early years (considered to be approximately 0–5 years) to the remainder of the child's life (Fonagy 1998; McCain & Mustard 1999). This highlights the value to students of the opportunity to develop an understanding of factors that contribute to or detract from such an environment, as well as to acquire knowledge of how, by adopting a partnership approach to working with families, nurses can facilitate a process of building on a family's strengths in the care of their infant, child and/or young person.

The location of the student may determine the range and acuity of clinical placements in child and adolescent healthcare that are available. For students located in regional areas, acute child and adolescent healthcare experience may be limited to general paediatrics, gained in a single ward designated for this specialty in a general hospital. On the other hand students located in a metropolitan area may have access to a tertiary level paediatric hospital offering a variety of neonatal, child and adolescent health experience. Within the bounds of service requirements, however, whether the student is located in a regional or metropolitan area, the opportunity for community-based experience in child and adolescent health is also likely to be available.

Preparing for the placement

Preparation for a placement in child and adolescent health includes the promotion of an understanding that children are not little adults. This realisation not only influences anatomical and physiological issues but also those relating to differences in expression of requirements in and responses to healthcare delivery. Examples of this include the facts that children express pain and distress, and interact with healthcare professionals, differently from adults. This emphasises the importance of including parents and family carers in all aspects of healthcare delivery in this specialty of nursing, because it is these carers who are most frequently best able to interpret the needs and responses of their child. Preparation for placement should also promote the student's knowledge of the legal requirements within which nurses (and other health professionals) practise, particularly those concerning child-protection legislation.

Challenges for the student

Particular challenges faced by the student during clinical placement in child and adolescent healthcare delivery relate to the need to communicate across the age range that the specialty encompasses, as well as with parents and families overall. Challenges for the student also frequently stem from the vulnerability and overall powerlessness of infants, children or young people, a vulnerability that may not just relate to the affect of health requirements, but also result from their family situation and their interaction with their families.

References

Fonagy P 1998 Prevention, the appropriate target of infant psychotherapy. Infant Mental Health Journal 19(2):124–150.

Harmon Hanson SM 2005 Family health care nursing: an Introduction. In SM Harmon Hanson, V Gedaly-Duff & J Rowe Kaakinen (eds), Family health care nursing, 3rd edn, pp 3–37. FA Davis, Philadelphia.

McCain M & Mustard JF 1999 Early years study: reversing the real brain drain. Ontario Children's Secretariat, Toronto.

Wong DL 1999 Whaley and Wong's nursing care of infants and children, 6th edn. Mosby, St Louis.

6.2 Community health nursing

Cheryle Morley
Interim Nurse Manager, Community Child
and Family Health Services, Primary Care and
Community Health Network, Sydney West Area
Health Service

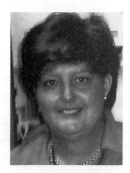

Bronwyn Warne
Cheryle Morley

Interim Nurse Manager, Community Chronic and
Complex Care Services Primary Care and
Community Health Network, Sydney West
Area Health Service

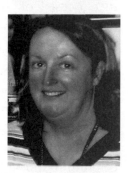

Bronwyn Warne

Overview of practice environment

Community nursing is a specialised clinical practice area where nurses are involved in the provision of healthcare to community-based clients outside of the acute hospital facilities. Services may be provided in the clients' homes, clinics, neighbourhood centres and schools. Generally nurses are based in community health centres and are part of a larger multidisciplinary team that covers a specific geographical area.

History of community nursing

Historically community nursing has been practised in many forms. The 'good wives' and 'witches' of the middle ages were perhaps early forms of community nurses, while in Australia the 'brown nurses', or Sisters of Charity, an order of nuns, established a visiting service to the poor and needy in 1838. A domiciliary nursing service began in Victoria in 1885, and in 1910, Lady Douglas, the wife of the then governor general, established the Bush Nursing Service (Burchill 1992, cited by Ward 1999).

The 1930s saw the introduction of baby health sisters and school nurses to effect change on the high rate of infant mortality and poor health of school children. This specialisation continued until the 1970s, when the generalist model of community nursing, often referred to as 'womb to tomb' or 'birth to death', was conceived as a service in 1972. The aim of this service was to provide healthcare that focused on health promotion, prevention of illness, school health screening, home nursing, early childhood health services and supportive services for clients at risk of health breakdown (O'Connor 1973, cited by Ward, 1999).

Following the acceptance and signing of the Alma Ata declaration by the Australian Government in Ottawa in 1978, and the consequent move by nurses to work within the framework of primary health care, the role, profile and range of skills required to practice as a community nurse have changed significantly in recent years (Ward 1999). The emphasis on early identification and intervention in child and family health services (as well as the increase in the ageing population and numbers of chronically ill) has resulted in huge demands on the generalist role of community nurses and hence the development of specialist roles (Kemp et al 2005).

The community environment as a learning experience

Placement in the community setting gives you a unique opportunity to observe and participate in nursing services provided for clients in their own environment, either at home, in clinics or in schools. The model of care is client-focused, with a holistic approach to assessment and intervention. In some areas the community nurse will be working with clients across the life span, while in other communities the demands on the generalist model has lead to the development of more specialised teams focusing on particular population groups, such as aged and chronic care, and child and family health.

Learning opportunities

It is expected that you will be working with a registered nurse or enrolled nurse for the duration of the clinical placement. During the placement you will have the opportunity to be involved in some hands-on work, but the specialised nature of the community nursing role limits this aspect and results in the clinical placement having a greater observational component for students than you may like.

There will be opportunities for you to explore one or many clinical specialty areas. These include child and family health nursing such as home visiting for families with newborn babies, audiometry, infant feeding and lactation, school screening and parenting education, as well as aged care, wound management, palliative care, continence and women's health services, and a number of allied health services that make up the larger multidisciplinary teams providing services in community health. You will benefit from discussion with practitioners in relation to the application of primary healthcare principles, recognising the alteration in balance of power when working with clients in their own environment and identifying networks and partnerships with other organisations and agencies that are core components of community health services (McDonald & Harris 2004).

For the placement to have the greatest value, you will need to have a good knowledge and understanding of the core principles of nursing practice. These include codes of conduct, ethics and accountability, legal aspects of care including consent for service, advocacy, infection control, documentation and confidentiality (client and staff). It is important that you recognise that these principles remain constant in all aspects of nursing practice, even though the work environment changes. Safety, security and manual handling have significant relevance in the community setting.

Preparing for the placement

You will need to discuss with your course/unit coordinator how your placement will be confirmed. In some situations the university undertakes all liaison, but at other times you may need to contact the nursing unit manager (NUM) yourself before you begin the placement. In most instances a student orientation package will be available on commencement, providing you with an overview of the service.

Generally, you will leave the community health centre or base in the morning and not return until later in the afternoon. As you will be away from the centre for most of the day, bring fluids to drink and make enquiries about the availability of food if you cannot bring it from home.

Challenges for students

Students have sometimes been challenged by the vast differences between community nursing and nursing in the acute sector. Community nursing can seem less exciting and isolated, and the time spent with one client once per week is hard to equate with the hospitalised client receiving constant contact over a whole shift. Another challenge relates to the perception of nurses having 'a lovely job just visiting new babies every day', especially when you may be confronted with the psychosocial risks and vulnerabilities that impact on some of the families community nurses work with. The shift in emphasis from hospital to community care because of increased cost of hospitalisation, decreased length of stay and early discharge means that nurses practising in the community have to manage more highly dependent and complex clients than they have done in the past (Kemp et al 2005). When nurses return to their base, paperwork is done and phone consultations and operational meetings take place. You will be encouraged to participate as you are able, but this time at the base also provides an opportunity to find out more about the clinical practice area, to observe other aspects of the service such as intake of referrals and to discuss services with other members of the interdisciplinary team.

Working with clients in their own environments means we need to accept that the client has the right to self-determination and that the community nurse develops the plan for care in collaboration with the client. Each client and her or his environment can be a learning situation; we acknowledge that people live in a variety of settings—from mansions to shipping containers with no electricity or running water. Some aspects of our work can also be confronting; debriefing with the nurse who you are working with is encouraged after visits, and the NUM is available to discuss and address any concerns and issues that you may have during the placement.

In some situations it may not be appropriate for you to accompany the community nurse on a visit. This could occur when a mother has postnatal depression or if the nurse is working with a family where there are child protection issues. Alternative arrangements will be made for you if this situation arises.

Community nursing as a career

Community nursing is an option for student nurses to consider for their future careers. Not only are there specialty areas of practice as previously outlined, there are also essential requirements for nurses entering this area of practice. Postgraduate experience and qualifications can be discussed during the placement, as well as the variety of specialties and career paths that are available for community nurses of the future.

Further reading

Centre for Health Equity Training, Research and Evaluation, University of New South Wales, <http://chetre.med.unsw.edu.au/>.
NSW Health, Planning better health: background information. Online. Available <http://www.health.nsw.gov.au/pubs/2004/pdf/pbh_booklet.pdf>.

Community health information

Federal: <http://www.health.gov.au>.
Australian Capital Territory: <http://www.health.act.gov.au>.
New South Wales: <http://www.health.nsw.gov.au>.
Northern Territory: <http://www.health.nt.gov.au>.
Queensland: <http://www.health.qld.gov.au>.
South Australia: <http://www.health.sa.gov.au>.
Victoria: <http://www.health.vic.gov.au>.
Western Australia: <http://www.health.wa.gov.au>.

References

Kemp LA, Comino EJ & Harris E 2005 Changes in community nursing in Australia. Journal of Advanced Nursing 49(2):307–314.
McDonald J & Harris E 2004 Guidelines: core functions and services for primary and community health services in NSW. Online. Available <http://chetre.med.unsw.edu.au/files/McDonald_J_(2004)_P&CH_Functions_&_Services_Guidelines.pdf>, 14 March 2006.
Ward D 1999 Master of Primary Health study guide. University Western Sydney, Penrith.

6.3 Critical care nursing

Jan Roche
Lecturer and Clinical Educator,
School of Nursing and Midwifery,
University of Newcastle

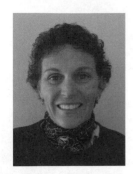

Jan Roche

Critical care nursing is practised in various settings, which include intensive care (ICU), high dependency (HDU), coronary care (CCU), and recovery/anaesthetics/operating theatres (OT). These areas are designed to provide total care to patients with overwhelming illness or injury on a one-to-one or one-to-two patient-to-nurse basis. Although the care is specialised and often uses the latest technology, the staff in these areas give complete basic nursing care and are highly skilled in assessment, allowing them to respond to emergency situations effectively.

Critical care areas offer the student nurse valuable learning opportunities. The ICU area has patients with multiple organ failure who often require artificial ventilation. These patients are constantly monitored. Regular observations of vital signs (including pulse, blood pressure, temperature and respiration) are designed to check the status of each of the patient's bodily systems. Head-to-toe assessment routinely includes checking a patient's neurological, cardiac and fluid balance status, as well as body alignment and skin integrity. Cardiac monitors and ventilators need to be checked regularly and the patient's pathology results reviewed. There are also focused observations for treatments including, but not limited to, underwater seal drains, intracranial pressure drains and haemodialysis. HDU patients are one step down from ICU patients. In this area, patients are not ventilated; however, they are still constantly monitored and assessed.

CCU is a specialised area for unstable cardiac patients. These patients are attached to cardiac monitors that are visible from the nurses' station.

The recovery/anaesthetics/OT patients range from the well person having an elective operation to the critically ill patient undergoing complex and life-saving procedures.

In all critical care areas, the opportunities for learning are enormous. The care ratio of one nurse to one or two patients gives you the opportunity to be involved in all aspects of total patient care as well as allowing you to work as part of an interdisciplinary healthcare team. Make the most of opportunities to learn about movement, chest physiotherapy, X-rays etc. The skills of airway management, cardiac rhythm interpretation and pain management are a normal part of practice. The advantage for you as a student is that a registered nurse with specialised knowledge of the area is there with you.

To really make the best of these opportunities you need to come prepared. Find out about the type of patients in the unit before your clinical placement. Review the pathophysiology for the common problems in the area. Look up the common treatments and medications. Arm yourself with as much knowledge as possible. Discuss your learning objectives with your mentor as well as your mentor's expectations of you.

There are many new and exciting situations in critical care. It is the difficult and sometimes sad cases where patients do not survive that are the most challenging. The critical care team all need debriefing after a death of a patient. Never be afraid to ask for help from the university and your mentor.

Critical care areas have different routines from general wards. Allow yourself time to adjust and learn the routine. Ask plenty of questions to clarify situations. A major concern of mentors is when students attempt nursing procedures without adequate understanding and skill.

Most importantly, enjoy the placement. Practise, practise, practise—because there will always be new things to learn in critical care nursing.

6.4 Day surgery nursing

Alison Anderson
Clinical Nurse Educator, Day Surgery Admission
Centre, Sydney Adventist Hospital

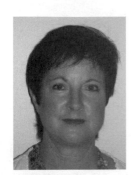

Alison Anderson

Day surgery continues to change and grow in Australia in keeping with advances in modern medicine. What was once considered a lengthy complex procedure may now be seen as a day case, and undergraduate students can take advantage of these opportunities in learning. Day surgery units (DSUs) may vary widely between different facilities, depending on whether they are publicly or privately funded, free-standing or part of a hospital campus, or specialty or general units. In all instances, they provide a great learning opportunity for maximising skills in assessment processes.

While each unit is very individualised, no matter how large or small it is or how many patients come through the doors each day, every nurse can be involved in, and be part of, a well-tuned team in which he or she will have an opportunity to share with patients their journey through a short and precise surgical experience. Patients benefit from reduced costs and recovery time, reduced time away from family and work, an easy transition from admission to anaesthetic/theatre and discharge, and the satisfaction of being in a caring environment especially tuned to safe discharge in a shortened time frame.

Nurses working in this environment benefit from the wide variety of experiences and learning opportunities gained from admission and assessment, operating theatre and recovery, through to discharge. Undergraduate nurses might be involved at all levels, which would provide an opportunity for them to sharpen skills in all areas. This will help them expand their knowledge base and understand the processes involved in assessment and decision-making, as well as allowing them to observe many surgical procedures and be involved in the recovery and discharge processes.

Learning opportunities

- An opportunity to be directly involved in ongoing education, including the use of written material, may suit the nurse who enjoys the wider interaction necessary between patients and their families.
- Day surgery units provide nurses with an opportunity to work closely with the patient and family in deciding appropriate patient care and outcomes.
- Excellent assessment in the preoperative stage prevents patients from having an adverse outcome during surgery. In day surgery units you will learn how to fully assess the patient and act on abnormal findings while understanding the needs of the specialty.
- You will have the opportunity to learn about new surgical procedures across all specialties. Some facilities include nurses in the operating theatre and recovery unit as well as in preoperative and discharge preparation.
- You will learn about anaesthetics used for day patients, why some patients have local blocks/anaesthetics or go home with continuous pumps, and what is it about day patient surgery that changes anaesthetic requirements.
- You can fine tune assessment skills for the management of postoperative pain, nausea and vomiting.
- You can gain knowledge of different wounds and how they can be managed at home by the day patient.
- You will develop personal skills in communication, prioritising work and working as part of a unique team.

Preparing for the placement

Before starting the placement, research the following:

- best practice guidelines for day surgery facilities
- current trends in anaesthetics for day patients, including local anaesthetic agents and blocks
- surgical procedures relevant to day surgery (e.g. gynaecology, orthopaedic, ENT, endoscopy, urology)
- nursing assessment and its application to the surgical patient
- discharge planning for the day patient

Challenges for students

- Depending on patient numbers in a given facility, students' experiences may vary widely. It would be helpful to find out what cases are done and what the facility offers patients and then to focus on one or two areas of interest.
- Some facilities that are day admission centres may have more than 80 patients attending in a day, which would challenge the student's ability to cope with variety and prioritising workloads.
- Moving from a pre-admission clinic, to admissions, to postoperative recovery may confuse students and leave them with a fragmented experience. Working in any one of those areas at a time will enhance the experience and provide for a more settled and worthwhile time.
- Staff may be under pressure, and a variety of healthcare professionals may be seen to come and go in the unit. This can be distracting; however, taken in context and with a well-trained mentor on hand, looking and learning can provide a positive experience.
- Tiredness will make it more difficult for the student to focus on the job. On a supernumerary placement, take time out to stay in tune with goals and learning outcomes, and discuss your needs with your mentor or clinical educator to ensure your experience is of the greatest value to you.

Helpful hints

- Ask lots of questions.
- Have a plan of what you want to learn and tell someone about it.
- Find out where you can get more information.
- Take notes.
- Read doctors' and hospital protocols and care plans/pathways.
- Be happy and attentive.
- Find out more about a specialty that interests you.
- Chose a patient (or two) to follow for a day.
- Remember: day surgery is the front door to your surgical experience. What you learn about assessment at all stages of the patient's journey through the facility should enhance your lifelong learning experience.

Nursing assessment case studies

Mr J, aged 35, is admitted to the day surgery unit for a knee arthroscopy. In clipping the knee to remove hair around the surgical site, the nurse notices a small, reddened graze with a weeping centre near the knee. On questioning the patient about this, he informs her that it was a result of a cycling accident two days ago. It is now a lot better than it has been and he has been treating it by painting it with Betadine four times a day. The nurse informs the attending medical officer, who comes to look at the knee and advises that the surgery must be postponed.

Postponing the procedure until the graze has healed reduces the risk of postoperative wound or bone infection, which would be increased if the surgery goes ahead. The nurse's assessment and subsequent intervention have saved the patient the embarrassment of having his procedure cancelled from the operating theatre list. Not proceeding with the set up of the theatre for this case saves the facility time and expense.

Mrs M, aged 84, is recovering in the postoperative area of the day surgery unit following colonoscopy. She complains of bloating and abdominal pain. The nurse obtains a clear understanding of the degree, type and location of the pain and following consultation with the RN decides to treat Mrs M with two paracetamol tablets and a cup of peppermint tea. Following this Mrs M is helped to the toilet, where she passes a lot of flatus and immediately feels a lot better. Half an hour later Mrs M's observations are within normal limits. She meets all the discharge criteria required by the facility, and is assisted to dress for discharge.

- Obtaining a clear history of postoperative pain enables the nurse to make decisions about management and care.
- Discussing the case with a senior nurse allows a team approach to treating and managing the postoperative patient and draws on the senior nurse's experience.
- By returning to assess the patient following an intervention, the nurse can determine if further treatment is necessary.
- Sending a patient home too soon from a day surgery unit may lead to an adverse outcome for the patient and family, and a negative experience.

Resource

Australian Day Surgery Nurse Association website: <http://www.adsna.info/index.html>.

6.5 Developmental disability nursing

Kristen Wiltshire
Nurse Learning and Development
Officer, Hunter Residences DADHC

Bill Learmonth
Manager Learning and
Development Officer,
Hunter Residences DADHC

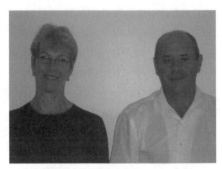

Kristen Wiltshire and Bill Learmonth

Developmental disability services provide services to people with a disability of any age in large residential and community settings. Both government and non-government disability services focus on supporting clients to lead valued, independent lives, with the opportunity to participate fully in the community.

Services provided are comprehensive and include nursing care for people with complex support needs in areas of multiple disability and behaviour intervention. The majority of clients in residential facilities are severely intellectually disabled adults with complex and concurrent disabilities. These disabilities may include sensory impairment, lack of mobility or altered mobility that is exacerbated by the normal ageing process, epilepsy or other medical conditions and/or challenging behaviour. People with an intellectual disability may suffer from a range of health issues faced by other people in the general community; however, their disability may put them at greater risk owing to difficulties associated with early identification and diagnosis. The role of nursing staff in recognising deviations from normal functioning in clients is vital. Some conditions such as epilepsy are more likely to be seen because of pre-existing conditions such as brain damage.

The complexity of the health needs of clients requires a coordinated and interdisciplinary approach by a team of health professionals. For some clients, the cause of their intellectual disability may result in many other associated health problems. For example, clients with Down syndrome are more likely to have cardiac and respiratory problems, thyroid disease, diabetes and coeliac disease.

It is important to uphold the rights of disabled people to make choices about the services they wish to be provided for them. Consent for medical procedures must be given by a 'person responsible', who is nominated by the guardianship tribunal. In emergency situations a medical practitioner can intervene if necessary.

There is usually a range of services available, including those provided by visiting specialists, who see clients with medical problems. These clients can be treated and monitored on site, but in some circumstances they will be referred to specialists in the general hospital system.

Many people with disabilities live in community homes and/or are cared for by families and will access a range of healthcare facilities, both private and public. It is an asset for nurses to develop experience in disability nursing in order to identify and provide nursing care when clients with disabilities present with their multiple health needs. In the general hospital system, a high percentage of medical and nursing staff may be inexperienced in dealing with people with intellectual or physical disabilities and their carers.

Learning opportunities

Disability services provide a microcosm of a whole range of learning opportunities. Students will have the opportunity to care for clients with disabilities and conditions that are rarely seen in the general public health system: for example, syndromes such as Retts, congenital rubella syndrome, Dandy Walker, cri-du-chat and cytomegalovirus.

The client population is also ageing and in some cases they are ageing more quickly than the normal community. This means that issues such as mobility, depression, anxiety, dementia, osteoporosis, diabetes, heart problems and cancer add to the complex nature of the care nurses need to provide.

Clients may exhibit 'challenging behaviour', which is behaviour that can interfere with the clients or staff carer's daily life experiences. Challenging behaviour is not an inevitable result of developmental disability, but it can contribute to social isolation and lack of opportunities for clients. A significant emphasis is placed on identifying clients' lifestyle needs to reduce the frequency of challenging behaviour and to enhance their lifestyle. Clients also have the opportunity to attend activity centres and participate in stimulating and diversional therapy.

Preparing for the placement

- Develop an awareness of the range of services available and the healthcare requirements of people with disabilities and their families.
- Develop an understanding of the *Disability Services Act* and Disability Services standards.
- Provide holistic nursing care on the basis of individual planning.

Challenges for students

The challenge for students will be to understand the complexity of the health needs of people with disabilities. As well as competing health needs, the clients have many disabilities that make providing care more difficult. Feeding, hydration and maintaining adequate nutrition is very important, as many clients with disabilities have dysphagia (difficulty swallowing). Meeting clients' mobility needs will often involve using a range of equipment. Many clients have limited or no verbal communication skills and rely on non-verbal communication such as gestures, sign language and augmentative communication devices. Verbal communication can also be limited to vocal sounds and/or limited vocabulary.

6.6 General practice nursing

Elizabeth J Halcomb
Senior Research Fellow, Centre for Applied
Nursing Research, Sydney South West Area
Health Service, and School of Nursing, College of
Health and Science, University of Western Sydney

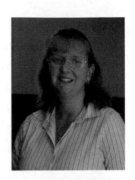

Elizabeth J Halcomb

General practices are an integral component of our health system, as they provide front-line management of health needs in the community. Although general practice receives significant public subsidy, it remains a private professional industry. This has important implications for the services that are provided and the accessibility of services to the community. Individual general practices in geographical areas have formed divisions of general practice to provide support (such as continuing education, professional support groups, divisional health programs), establish links with other healthcare agencies (for example, acute hospitals, community care providers) and act as a representative body for general practice (Commonwealth Department of Health and Aged Care 2005). In 2005, 122 divisions existed across Australia.

Currently, around 8 per cent of people in Australia visit a general practitioner annually, with increased use of the service commonly seen in those of advanced age or chronic illness and complex health needs (Britt et al 2004; Commonwealth Department of Health and Family Services 2000; Macklin 1992; New South Wales Department of Health 2002). While practice nursing is a well-developed specialty area in the United Kingdom and New Zealand, it remains largely in its infancy in Australia. Although nurses have worked in Australian general practice for many years, it is only recently that the number of nurses has increased and their roles have developed (Halcomb et al 2005). This has largely been the result of federal government initiatives that have provided additional funding for the employment of practice nurses and allowed practice nurses to claim Medicare items for certain procedures (Halcomb et al 2005).

Learning opportunities

General practice is an important learning environment for nursing students, as it provides an opportunity to participate actively in the delivery of primary care. In turn, this allows the nurse to develop an appreciation for the complexity of health issues facing the community and of the health services available in the general practice setting. The experience will assist in broadening the outlook not only of those students wishing to pursue a career in community or practice nursing, but also of those seeking employment in the acute sector. Practice nursing is an emerging nursing field in Australia and it is an exciting time to be introduced this specialty, as there are significant opportunities to contribute to the health of the community, as well as to develop a clinical career pathway.

Preparing for the placement

Unlike the acute care setting, the roles of clinicians in the general practice team and the daily routine can vary significantly from practice to practice. This is due to a number of factors, including the personal preferences of the general practitioner (GP), the skill level of the practice nurse, other services available in the local community (such as private pathology laboratory) or practice (such as allied health), and the resources of the practice. To gain the most from your placement, you need to have a clear understanding of how the practice nurse and individual GPs collaborate to provide care and the usual routine of the nurse within the practice.

The demographics of the local community and, more specifically, of the practice population will have an impact upon the nature of clinical presentations in the general practice you visit. Having an understanding of the local community and any specific health issues that it faces will assist you to prepare for placement.

Challenges for the student

It is likely that you will be exposed to a wide range of clinical presentations, from acute conditions and acute exacerbations of chronic illness, to preventative activities (for example, pap smears, immunisations, lifestyle advice) and chronic disease management. Such encounters will allow you to consolidate a range of clinical skills from communication and counselling to physical assessment, wound dressing, assisting the GP with minor surgery, venepuncture and measurement of physical parameters (for example, electrocardiograms, peak flow meter, blood pressure assessment). It is this diversity and the often fast pace that will probably present you with the greatest challenge during your placement.

A characteristic of practice nursing that attracts many to the specialty is the relative autonomy that the nurse has in providing care. In many practices, a single nurse may be working in a practice at a time. This represents a challenge to nurses as it is often associated with professional isolation. It is for this reason that professional networks have been established in many divisions of general practice to provide support and continuing education. For you the student, however, it may be challenging to work in this model with a small group of nurse mentors for support. Before beginning a placement in general practice, you should be aware of key contacts both internal and external to the practice that can provide support should it be required.

References

Britt H, Miller GC, Charles J et al 2004 General practice activity in the states and territories of Australia 1998–2003 (GP Series no. 15, AIHW Cat No GEP 15). General Practice Statistics and Classification Unit, University of Sydney and Australian Institute of Health and Welfare, Canberra.

Commonwealth Department of Health and Aged Care 2005 General practice in Australia: 2004. Australian Government Printing Service, Canberra.

Commonwealth Department of Health and Family Services 2000 General practice in Australia: 2000. Australian Government Printing Service, Canberra.

Halcomb E, Davidson P, Daly J et al 2005 Nursing in Australian general practice: directives and perspectives. Australian Health Review 29(2):156–166.

Macklin J 1992 The future of general practice (National Health Strategy Issues Paper no. 3). Department of Health, Housing and Community Services Canberra.

New South Wales Department of Health 2002 Strengthening health care in the community. NSW action plan for health (bulletin no. 7). NSW Department of Health, Sydney.

6.7 Indigenous health nursing

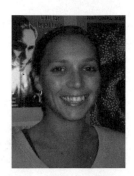

Rebekah O'Reilly
Community Nurse, Daruk Aboriginal Community
Controlled Medical Service Co-op Ltd

Rebekah O'Reilly

Aboriginal community-controlled health organisations (ACCHOs), also known as Aboriginal medical services, have an important role to play in combatting the high rates of ill health and early death in Aboriginal communities. An Aboriginal board of directors, elected by the Aboriginal community, governs each Aboriginal medical service. Aboriginal medical services aim to provide culturally appropriate, holistic primary healthcare services targeted to the needs of their local Aboriginal community.

Using a 'whole of life' approach, health services are provided by Aboriginal health workers, nurses and doctors, and include specialised services for children, the aged and those with disabilities. This may be through centre-based clinical care, home visits, health promotion and/or preventative activities. Many health issues—such as men's and women's health, antenatal care, mental health, oral health and substance misuse—are treated within Aboriginal medical services.

Placements in community settings such as Aboriginal medical services are important for students. They help students gain an understanding of how different community services are integrated into the local community and interact with other community services in the area. Most families and individuals make use of more than one community service. Knowing what each service provides gives the student a broader knowledge of holistic healthcare outside the hospital.

Students who have the opportunity to spend time in an Aboriginal medical service will enhance many skills. They will learn the various ways to deliver healthcare to Aboriginal people according to age, socioeconomic status and education level. Effective communication is a key factor in working in the community, as is time management. For example, what was expected to be a 'short home visit' could become much longer once the nurse finds she or he needs to treat more than one person living in a large, shared household.

Before beginning a placement in an Aboriginal medical service, students should have some understanding and knowledge of Indigenous culture and the principles of cultural safety. It can take time to build up the trust required to work effectively with the community. For example, Aboriginal clients may ask a lot of questions of new nurses before they will divulge any information, and home visits may be carried out at the front door until people are comfortable enough to invite you in. Before attending a clinical placement in an Aboriginal medical centre, students should be aware of the history of Aboriginal people, including the 'stolen generations', and the effect the past still has on Aboriginal communities today. Most importantly, a sound knowledge of the health issues affecting Aboriginal people will help those students considering a career in Aboriginal medical services to understand the challenges and rewards of working in such a dynamic and interesting work environment.

6.8 Justice health nursing

Petra Bell
Nurse Educator, Justice Health, Long Bay
Correctional Centre, Sydney

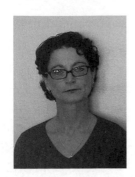

Petra Bell

Across Australia, different institutions support the health needs of incarcerated persons and students are encouraged to investigate the types of services that are offered to these patients. The term 'justice health' is commonly used in New South Wales, replacing 'corrections health' in 2004. Elsewhere in Australia, students may come across other terms such as correctional health, prison services healthcare, prison health, forensic medical services, forensic mental health or forensic care. Within this specialised area of healthcare, clinical placements may be available to nursing students.

In New South Wales, the healthcare of incarcerated persons is the responsibility of Justice Health, a statutory health corporation constituted under the *NSW Health Services Act 1997* to care for a health community that is unique in New South Wales, consisting of more than 21,500 inmates annually. The challenges that face staff working in this and similar environments are many. Some of them include the remote geographical location of clinics, the high turnover and frequent relocation of patients, and the need to develop and provide appropriate services for both long-term and very short-term inmates and detainees.

A patient's health needs in such an environment are far greater than those of the general community, as health is often not a priority before incarceration. On reception into the correctional system, a comprehensive health needs assessment is completed for each patient. Key issues for staff to consider include the following:

- a high incidence of serious mental illness
- drug- and alcohol-dependent patients who require management of detoxification on reception
- a high prevalence of hepatitis C
- the prevention of self-harm and suicide, and effective management of incidents and attempts
- meeting the health needs of female patients, whose numbers have increased by 45 per cent since 1998
- health promotion and harm minimisation

Nursing staff work closely in partnership with other government departments, such as Corrective Services, which means that nurses can provide appropriate health services within a secure correctional environment.

Learning opportunities

Learning experiences may fall into a number of health service areas.

Mental health

The student may be involved in the following areas:

- ambulatory patient services, including visiting psychiatrists, registered mental health nurses, crisis and multidisciplinary risk intervention teams
- mental health screening
- managing patients with acute psychiatric illnesses
- undertaking forensic history and conducting psychiatric evaluations as requested by the magistrate

Community/primary health

A community approach is provided for patients in correctional centres. The desirable primary health model is holistic, encompassing population health, drug and alcohol, and mental health and focusing on chronic and complex conditions.

Population health

Public/sexual health nurses work autonomously in clinic settings. There is no direct equivalent to the role of a public/sexual health nurse in the community. It is a hybrid role with a strong focus on harm minimisation.

Drug and alcohol

These services are vitally important in a correctional environment owing to the high rate of substance use by patients. Patients who are opiate dependent (e.g. methadone and buprenorphine) are offered a range of pharmacotherapy. In partnership with the National Drug and Alcohol Research Centre and the Department of Corrective Services, a naltrexone trial has also been established. Inpatient detoxification services are also offered to patients.

Women's health

Women's health centres offer all the above services, with some centres offering antenatal care and a mother and children's program. This type of nursing is not only a learning experience but also a life-altering experience.

Challenges for the student

In this type of placement students may encounter a variety of challenges:

- working in a interdisciplinary environment
- working within the walls of a correctional facility
- working within the judicial system and observing the effects it has on our patients
- observing the effects of incarceration on mentally ill patients
- addressing the bio-psychosocial needs of patients
- developing an awareness of the limited education and life skills of the majority of patients

Security is paramount in this environment and criminal record clearances are mandatory. Patient access is totally reliant on correctional officers and all patient treatment must be delivered within sight or sound of a correctional officer. Other security measures include limitations on what personal items may be taken into facilities. Students must carry their educational institution's identity card at all times, sign a privacy form and have an awareness of both professional and personal boundary issues.

Preparing for the placement

If you are interested in this type of placement, it is advisable to read information provided by the facility to your educational institution before starting your placement. Owing to the unique environment, this type of facility will have its own clinical educators or staff to support students, and you will be encouraged to reflect on your views and beliefs regarding offenders. Patients encountered on these placements are incarcerated as punishment for their crimes, but retain a right to healthcare, which Justice Health (and specialised health service agencies in other states and territories of Australia) delivers.

6.9 Medical nursing

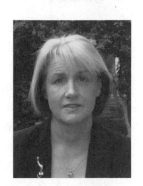

Kristina Roberts

Assistant Director of Nursing, Auburn Hospital,
Sydney West Area Health Service

Kristina Roberts

The acute care hospital comprises diverse care environments for inpatient services (Crisp & Taylor 2001). The medical unit is one such unit that requires nurses to have sound skills and knowledge to practice in this core clinical area. While multiple models of nursing care may be used in medical units by nurses across Australia, essentially it is the nature of the patient's medical condition (disease, illness and treatment requirements) and the hospital's bed management system that will determine if patients will be admitted to the medical ward. Nursing care is formulated around assessment that assumes multiple causes for the problems that are being experienced by the patient (see *Mosby's Dictionary of Medicine, Nursing and Health Professions*, 2006).

Medical nursing is a challenging and rewarding opportunity for all students. In the learning environment of the ward, students will be presented with countless opportunities to gain clinically based experiences and to practise nursing skills. The work is demanding both physically and emotionally, and within your student role you will be constantly drawing not only on the knowledge and skills you have gained theoretically, but on the 'people' skills you have been building on throughout your life. As well as your nursing skills, the patients on the medical ward need your caring, understanding and humanity.

The patients you will be nursing will come from all walks of life. Some of these patients will be chronically ill and used to frequent hospital stays; others will be just finding out that they face serious, life-threatening problems requiring multiple admissions to hospital to undergo unpleasant treatments. You will be caring for patients across the age continuum, from the very young to the very old. Some of these patients will have complex problems; others will have physical illnesses that are complicated by mental health issues. You will experience a wide range of patient behaviours and human emotions necessitating your patience and understanding.

You can expect to learn a great deal about your patients and their medical conditions during a placement on a medical ward. You will learn about medical conditions such as metabolic conditions (for example, diabetes), cardiac and respiratory disorders (for example, asthma), cerebral vascular disease, cancer, disorders associated with aging and much more. You will gain valuable experience handling a wide range of medications and treatment regimens and will have the opportunity to perfect your nursing skills, including observation, assessment and patient care. An important experience will be learning how to function as a valuable member of the interdisciplinary healthcare team, working not only with nurses and doctors, but also with physiotherapists, occupational therapists, speech pathologists, social workers and others.

To prepare yourself for this exciting and valuable learning experience, reread your notes, journal articles and textbooks about common patient conditions such as diabetes, heart disease, and respiratory and common blood disorders. Find out what you can about the common drugs used in the treatment of these disorders and their side effects, and the precautions the nurse administering these medications should take. Before your placement, practise assessment skills such as observing vital signs and using the glucometer. Be comfortable with the handling of intravenous lines and setting drip rates. Keep in mind that the more confident and dextrous you are during your practice sessions, the more receptive to learning you will be and the safer your patients will feel in the ward setting.

A variety of nursing skills are undertaken to provide care for patients in the medical ward. These patient requirements will provide you with the opportunity to practise your nursing skills. Remember that nursing is always patient-centred. The majority of nursing skills you will perform for patient care can be undertaken in more than one way, requiring you to adjust your technique to suit the individual patient and yet still adhere to principles of practice (Crisp and Taylor 2001).

Once you are on the ward, participate; become involved with the patients and the staff. Always be punctual, listen to handover, ask questions, use the resource material on the ward to broaden your knowledge and be ready to learn. Maximum learning opportunities come about when you work with your assigned nurse undertaking patient care. Offer your assistance; show that you are enthusiastic and that you want to learn. Medical ward nurses want to teach, and many nurses can remember what it was like to be a student. They value your contribution as a part of their team.

Medical nursing is challenging; it can be physically and emotionally demanding, yet it can also be very rewarding. Many of your patients will be long-term, chronically ill people looking to you for care and guidance. Some patients will be facing a crisis in their lives and they may turn to you for support. You will finish each shift tired but satisfied that you have made a difference to someone who needed you. If you are prepared to become involved, to participate and to show your enthusiasm, you will feel the satisfaction that comes with being a valued team member.

Good luck and enjoy your nursing.

Reference

Crisp J & Taylor C (eds) 2001 Potter and Perry's fundamentals of nursing. Mosby, Sydney.

6.10 Mental health nursing

Mike Hazelton
Head of School, Professor of Mental Health
Nursing, School of Nursing and Midwifery,
University of Newcastle and Hunter Mental Health

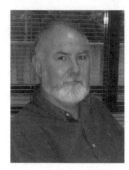

Professor Mike Hazelton

Mental health nursing is a speciality area of nursing and requires high levels of skill and knowledge to practise effectively. The users of mental health services are among the most vulnerable client groups in the healthcare system. In addition, many people admitted to institutional mental health facilities may have been legally compelled to undergo assessment and treatment. Even those receiving care in the community may be subject to community treatment orders requiring adherence to treatment regimens such as antipsychotic medication (Morrall & Hazelton 2004).

The existence of mental health nursing as a specialty should not be taken to imply that nurses working in other areas of healthcare will not come into contact with people suffering from severe mental health problems and disorders. Indeed, it is well known that specialist mental health services deal with only a minority of people in this client group (World Health Organization 2001). It is thus important that all nurses:

- can recognise the various forms of mental disorder.
- have sufficient interpersonal skills to be able to engage with and support people displaying the various forms of disturbance and distress associated with mental illness.
- are able to make appropriate judgments regarding the need to liaise with and/or refer to specialist mental health services.

- are familiar with the legal framework within which mental health care is provided.
- have a good understanding of available treatment options (Clinton et al 2001; Hazelton & Clinton 2001).

In addition to these basic knowledge and skill requirements, two crucial attitudinal considerations can be identified. First, students should be given the opportunity to develop an understanding of what it is like to experience mental illness from the perspective of mentally ill people and of those who live with them. The most effective way of providing this is to ensure meaningful input into the nursing curriculum by people who have been the users of mental health services and their close family members (Hazelton & Clinton 2001). Nowadays such people are readily available in most parts of the country and can be accessed via the local public mental health service. Second, nursing education in the mental health area should stress the importance of maintaining therapeutic optimism. Mental illness has long been associated with suboptimal care and ineffective treatments. However, given the availability of a wide range of treatments with demonstrated effectiveness, even the most severe disorders, such as schizophrenia or borderline personality disorder, can be approached with the expectation of good prospects for recovery (Fonagy & Bateman 2006).

Given the points raised above, the mental health practice environment may range from acute inpatient facilities (usually located in the grounds of general hospitals, but sometimes remaining as stand-alone psychiatric hospitals) to services located entirely in the community (either as walk-in community mental health clinics or as mobile round-the-clock community mental health teams providing outreach to clients in their places of residence). In relation to the organisation of clinical placements, wherever possible it would be desirable for students to experience mental health care in both institutional and community contexts, as engaging with service users in their own homes can be a very different experience from doing so in an acute inpatient facility. In particular, the capacity of many people to live meaningful lives in the community, despite ongoing high levels of psychiatric disability, can be a profoundly enlightening and humbling experience for health professionals.

Learning opportunities

In principle, all mental health services should be considered as providing sound learning opportunities. Whether this eventuates will depend on the extent of preparation and support provided by the responsible teaching staff, the preparation and commitment of students, and the support and enthusiasm of the staff receiving the students. At the very least, students should:

- familiarise themselves with the facilities and services to be involved in the clinical placement.
- become familiar with the range of learning experiences likely to be encountered in mental health services.
- access learning support material and resources provided.
- develop clearly specified learning objectives for the placement and communicate these to staff in the participating mental health services.
- become involved in the feedback and debriefing opportunities for students, both during and following completion of the clinical placement.
- develop and refine their interpersonal skills to be able to effectively engage with and support a person who is disturbed and/or distressed.

Preparing for the placement

For students to gain maximum benefit from clinical placements in mental health facilities it is important that they undertake background reading on the causes, clinical manifestations, treatments and treatment outcomes of mental health problems and disorders, focusing especially on the important contributions nurses make in this area of healthcare. In addition, it is crucial that students explore and critique their own assumptions regarding mental illness, with particular emphasis on ideas and beliefs that might be stigmatising and discriminatory.

Many students are understandably apprehensive about undertaking a clinical placement in mental health services (Farrell & Carr 1996) and, as the preceding discussion implies, students undertaking clinical placements in mental health settings face numerous challenges. These can range from initial apprehension associated with undertaking a placement in a service setting likely to be different from previous placements, to struggling to find much that is 'nursing' in what seems to be custodial work in inpatient settings, to concerns regarding personal safety. The skills and knowledge of mental health staff will be one of the most powerful resources and greatest supports available to students on placement.

References

Clinton M, du Boulay S, Hazelton M et al 2001 Mental health nursing education and the labour force: literature review. In National Review of Nursing Education 2002. Commonwealth of Australia, Canberra.

Farrell G & Carr J 1996 Who cares for the mentally ill? Theory and practice hours with a 'mental illness' focus in nursing curricula in Australian universities. Australian and New Zealand Journal of Mental health Nursing 5:77–83.

Fonagy P & Bateman A 2006 Progress in the treatment of borderline personality disorder. British Journal of Psychiatry 188:1–3.

Hazelton M & Clinton M 2001 Mental health consumers or citizens with mental health problems? In S. Henderson & A. Petersen (eds), Consuming health: the commodification of health care, pp 88–101. Routledge, London.

Morrall P & Hazelton M 2004 Mental health: global policies and human rights. Whurr Publishers, London.

World Health Organization 2001 The world health report 2001—mental health: new understanding, new hope. World Health Organization, Geneva.

6.11 Midwifery

Nita Purcal

Head of Program, Midwifery, School of Nursing,

College of Health and Science, University of Western Sydney

The practice environment

Maternity care is provided by midwives, who are health professionals skilled in offering holistic care to women from conception through the antenatal period, labour, birth and postnatal period up to and including six weeks post-delivery. It is different from other types of healthcare, as it is delivered to predominantly healthy women with a major emphasis on health promotion and health maintenance. Midwives play an important role in promoting health, detecting complications during pregnancy, labour and the postnatal period. They are skilled to carry out emergency measures and procure medical assistance.

In the context of maternity services in Australia, most women attend standard care in local hospitals. Following delivery, the practice of early discharge of well women and their babies is encouraged, and a follow-up home visiting service based on need is provided from the hospital. Specialist medical services are available in maternity units, but tend to be concentrated in larger referral hospitals. This may mean the transfer of a woman or a newborn baby with complications from a district hospital to a larger centre.

Midwives aim to offer women continuity of care models such as midwife-run clinics, team midwifery, birth centre care and some community birthing services.

There is a major emphasis on women having choice in the services provided, in being well informed about the care they receive, and being actively involved in decisions that affect the care they receive.

The maternity environment as a learning experience

The maternity environment demonstrates to the student nurse the high level of professional care required and available to women who are experiencing a normal biological function. Further, it shows how expediently other resources and services are implemented if complications arise, to ensure that risk factors are dealt with promptly.

Physical care is often seen to be the major function of maternity care, but the psychosocial, cultural, spiritual and educational aspects are attended to with equal importance. For example, the education process prepares couples for labour, birth, the postnatal period, care of the newborn baby and early parenting. The student will observe the supportive and educative role provided by midwives to assist women in self-care throughout pregnancy and birth, and the care of their newborn.

Students should understand that not all women have the same outcome. Stillbirth and neonatal death is a reality for some, in spite of the expert services available. Counselling and support services for all involved are therefore vital in these circumstances.

Upon discharge from hospital, all women are provided with local community contact numbers and support groups to assist and support them with newborn and infant care as well as with the challenging role of being a new parent. Health promotion and maintenance is important for the newborn, and mothers will receive information on most health services, including immunisation schedules.

Learning opportunities

Antenatal

Antenatally, the health and wellbeing of the woman and the developing fetus is paramount, with emphasis on nutrition, lifestyle and health-promoting behaviours. Learning opportunities include:

- observing screening processes for medical complications such as hypertension, glucose intolerance and infections.

- understanding how preparation for labour classes assist couples to plan for the forthcoming labour noting what they include in a birth plan and how the classes show them how to benefit from a labour support person.
- observing the importance attached to fetal wellbeing and how this is highlighted in each antenatal visit with noninvasive methods of screening, such as auscultation of the heart rate and advice to the mother on how to monitor fetal movements between clinic visits.

Birth

The birthing process dominates the thoughts of expectant couples to the extent that they give little attention at that stage to the lifelong role of being a parent. In the birthing units close observations of some labours will alert the student to the physiology of labour and how this differs between women, as well as the tolerance and experience of pain. For example, there will be women who have 'short' labours of a few hours, while others will labour for 10 hours or more. The role of the midwife and labour support person is one of physical and psychological support.

Pain in labour is a clinical sign of progress and women have different levels of tolerance and coping. Strong painful contractions are needed to move the fetus through the birth canal. Therefore, physiological pain is an expectation of labour. Non-pharmacological pain relief such as massage, position, warm showers and breathing techniques are offered to women. Medications are used with caution and only after a physical assessment of the progress of labour. Most medications used will cross the placenta and affect the fetus.

Birthing the baby requires maternal effort, but the rewards are profound, and the baby's first cry receives an emotional response from all those present. Delivery of the placenta and membranes includes the ritual inspection to ensure there are no retained products that could interfere with involution of the uterus. Note the detailed documentation of the entire birthing process and the identification requirements of the newborn.

Postnatal

The postnatal period includes care of the mother and her newborn, as the first 24 hours are a critical recovery period for the mother and one of extrauterine adaptation for the baby. In general, the care is holistic and the baby will room-in with mother. Monitoring of vital signs, physical assessment and involution of the uterus, lactation advice and support of breastfeeding will be just some of the care given to the mother. The baby requires physical assessment, observation and documentation of vital signs, feeding behaviour and excretory functions.

The psychosocial needs of the postnatal woman are important and the student will observe that midwives devote time to encouraging women to debrief their birth experience. Midwives encourage women to develop an early and long-lasting relationship with their babies by promoting rooming-in, education and support. Observe the behaviours and rituals practised by some mothers that are based on cultural traditions—for example, some Asian women delay breastfeeding.

Preparing for the placement

Students who plan their placements will be rewarded with a very professional educational and clinical experience.

Before starting the placement, read about maternity care and make some notes on the following:

- the purpose of antenatal care
- the stages of labour
- the differences between a natural birth and an operative delivery
- the purpose of postnatal care
- rationales for women having a hospital stay after birthing
- the need for some specialist services

Listen to birth stories from family and friends, and map some of their experiences to gain insight into what you can expect.

Review the objectives of the placement and try to link these to the clinical areas of the rotation.

Staying focused

Plan relevant objectives on a daily basis and avoid wandering around without a purpose. Review the objectives mid-placement with the clinical educator to ensure you are meeting the essential clinical experience of the placement.

Be aware that maternity services promote women participating in their own care. When on placement, observe how they do this and learn from them how they put together a plan for pregnancy and birth.

Students may experience a feeling of inadequacy and being overwhelmed by the clinical environment. This is a common feeling among students whether they are undergraduate or postgraduate. Be guided by your clinical educator and buddy-up with a midwife who will tell you what he or she is doing and why, and who will have most of the answers to your questions.

Reflect on one day at a time in preparation for the next day, be realistic and don't expect too much of yourself. Identify and explore challenges during your placement in maternity.

Challenges for the student

Organisation and planning

Some clinical areas, such as the antenatal clinic and postnatal ward, may strike you as being in chaos and very disorganised. Don't despair; the team leader is very proficient in ensuring women's needs are being met. Just prepare yourself to expect some degree of chaos, especially in the postnatal area where there are three main activities in the ward: women wanting physical care and assistance, others preparing for discharge, and a queue of women and babies emerging from the birthing unit and waiting on trolleys to be admitted.

Labour and birth

Your first experience of labouring women may be confronting: you may react to the physical appearance of the woman in labour, nudity and even the noises she may make. Expect to be on a steep learning curve and reflect on what you have read about the physical, psychosocial, spiritual and cultural aspects of labour.

One can never be adequately prepared for witnessing birth, as it is such an emotional journey for some; a few tissues in your pocket may help.

Complications

Obstetric and medical problems can occur in pregnancy, labour, birth and the postnatal period. An awareness of some of the complex situations that require medical intervention will confirm the importance of monitoring and early intervention to ensure good outcomes. Experience in the clinical area will challenge your need to learn more about the assessment, diagnosis and management.

Cultural sensitivity

Being culturally sensitive is as important as being competent in delivering physical care. Women and their family support members may require extra care based on needs such as bridging the language and religious barriers.

Loss and grief

Loss in broad terms may mean a woman's lost opportunity for something she had planned to gain from her pregnancy and birth or postnatal experience. For example, she may have planned a pharmacologically free labour, but have succumbed to medication; she may have wanted a natural birth but had to have an operative delivery because of fetal complications; or maybe she chose formula to feed her baby because of overwhelming difficulties with breastfeeding. The sense of loss women feel can be helped by providing an opportunity for debriefing.

The loss of a baby or mother in maternity care is rare, but is felt intensely by family and attending staff.

Conclusion

A placement in maternity care is challenging and rewarding. To witness the process is an amazing experience that will enhance your personal and professional development and enable you to reflect on natural and complex situations as you develop as a nurse.

6.12 Occupational health nursing

Judith Carlisle
Occupational Health Nurse Coordinator, Coal
Services Health, New South Wales

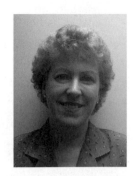

Judith Carlisle

Occupational health nurses (OHNs) play a key role in implementing all activities designed to promote the health of the worker. The precise duties of the OHN are tailored according to individual industry needs, and students undertaking placements with the OHN in industry will be exposed to a variety of health promotion activities.

According to Matilda Babbitz (1992), Executive Director, American Association of Occupational Health Nurses, OHN duties are varied. They include finding out workers' individual health needs, identifying industry hazards and their potential for harm, and understanding the relationship between illness and injury in the working environment. OHNs also need to establish professional standards consistent with company policy. The OHN needs to be autonomous and independent, self-directed and self-motivated in order to provide a diverse range of occupational health services to industry.

In general, the OHN may perform some of the following functions:

- Assist in general administration, maintenance and arrangement of health facilities.
- Provide for emergency and primary treatment of accidents and illnesses.
- Assist with pre-placement and other health surveillance.
- Arrange follow-up treatment, where indicated, including health supervision of employees returning to work following illness.
- Refer workers to general community agencies for help as necessary.

- Assist in general preventative health measures, adopting evidence-based practice.
- Provide health education and counselling.
- Assist in supervision of plant hygiene and accident prevention.
- Provide advice to management on specific health issues.
- Assist in designing and implementing workplace strategies for health surveillance and risk management.
- Assist in identifying health risks and use the evidence to design hygiene and wellness programs.

The OHN's role in health surveillance includes pre-placement health assessments, which are normally conducted before a person takes up a new position, when a worker transfers between sites and periodically to establish baseline data that allow deviations from normal health to be detected at an early stage. The purpose of the pre-placement assessment is to identify health conditions that may increase the health and safety risk to the client or to others in the workplace. The health assessment process involves recording a health history, conducting a series of tests and then analysing objective and subjective data to agree on the worker's ability to work safely, usually in consultation with an occupational physician.

Preparing for the placement

Reading in the following areas before placement will enhance the learning experience:

- the association between health assessment of individuals and health promotion
- occupational health risks relevant to the specific industrial group
- the nursing methods used to assess coronary artery risk factors and overnutrition
- the range of symptoms experienced by individuals with noise-induced hearing loss and the social impact of these symptoms

Learning opportunities

An occupational health placement will help students develop an understanding of the medical conditions likely to be encountered in the working population of the particular industry. They will also participate in clinical assessment and observe occupational health nursing practice. The placement may provide the opportunity to do some of the following: recording occupational and health history; measuring height, weight and BMI; performing urinalysis; testing visual acuity, including colour perception; audiometry; spirometry; alcohol and other drug testing; and observing physical examination, including a musculoskeletal assessment.

Students will also develop skills to identify general health, coronary artery and occupational health risks according to medical standards, participate in fitness-to-work and immunisation programs, and conduct literature searches to support evidence-based occupational health and safety practice.

Specifically, a student undertaking this type of placement will have the opportunity to do the following:

- Interview clients to record an occupational and health history.
- Perform clinical tests according to guidelines.
- Provide clients with feedback on findings during the health assessment process.
- Provide effective and meaningful health information aimed at health promotion.
- Work with a diverse team of health professionals.
- Identify individual occupational health and safety risk factors requiring further intervention to support fitness to work.

Reference

Babbitz M 1992 Approaching the 21st century. Congressional agenda for health care and occupational health. American Association of Occupational Health Nurses 40(1):12–16.

6.13 Older person nursing

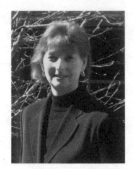

Tina Koch
Professor of Nursing (Older Person Care),
School of Nursing and Midwifery,
Faculty of Health, University of Newcastle

Professor Tina Koch

Who is old?

In 1999 the International Year of the Older Person declared that people are not aged, elderly of even old, merely older. However, the term 'older person' is generally used to refer to people who are aged 65 and over. In 2001 there were 2,370,878 people in Australia who were aged 65 and over, and this population is growing. It is known that this population includes a diversity of backgrounds and ages. This means that people included in this group are far from homogenous; they have a variety of lifestyles, living arrangements, family circumstances and cultural, social and religious practices. Such diversity means considering each person as an individual.

What is it like to have lived 100 years? What, in the opinion of centenarians, has contributed to their longevity? Is it important to manage stress well in order to live a long time? These were a few of the interview questions posed to 24 Australian centenarians (Koch et al 2005). In the interviews, the centenarians revealed that they did not think of themselves as old. Their stories were fascinating, showing their response to loss, their adaptability, their engagement and social connectedness, their strong religious beliefs and, without fail, their sense of humour. Their participation in volunteer activities, shared history of hard work and subsequent rejection of idleness add new insights into the emerging understanding of what makes a life meaningful. There is great diversity among these older people; their accounts of their health in the context of their lives reveal that there are no 'secrets' for longevity and no stereotypes.

It is important to remember the diversity that exists among older people and to invite them to tell their personal stories. Listen to the older person. The consequence of not listening and not treating the person as an individual places you at risk of stereotyping them. Viewing older people as sterotypes can profoundly affect the way they are perceived and consequently treated. Three of the most pervasive stereotypical views of ageing are that older people are physically incapable, mentally incapable and intellectually frail, and this has implications for their care. When this stereotyped perspective is adopted, the older person is seen as one whose improvement is unlikely, which suggests that maintaining the status quo is all that can be achieved. A picture emerges of a mentally frail and physically incapable human being who is not able to make a decision.

Combined with negative stereotyping, the biomedical construction of ageing has important implications for the way in which healthcare professionals view older people, and also the way in which ageism is perpetuated in the wider community. The biology of the ageing process is popularly perceived to justify beliefs about age. This perception of health has a narrow focus on pathological processes affecting parts of the body rather than on the whole person, and has tended to confirm a construct of ageing as a time of decay and decline.

The biomedical construct has almost exclusively been concerned with charting degenerative, as opposed to adaptive and developmental, progress. Central to this image is that the human machine grinds to a halt when parts wear out and that there is an increasing need for maintenance. Within this pathological perspective, health is measured in terms of the relative malfunctioning of the machinery that is the human body. Acute care delivery, with its focus on individual organic pathology and intervention, has become a powerful and pervasive force in the definition and treatment of ageing. Using the metaphor of the machine, the machine body can be entered, studied and tampered with in order to be repaired. The body becomes an object of inquiry, and the person as an individual fades into the background and becomes a biomedical object susceptible to interventions. It is suggested that this view in healthcare has been significant in determining ageist attitudes. In addition, the pathological model puts helpers in a superior position and those they help in an inferior position. To be helped or be in need of help means to be seen as incompetent, wrong, hapless, helpless or stupid. Being helped produces categories and labels for older people that limit possibilities for intervention and reduce the understanding healthcare professionals may develop, denying the person's history and personal meanings.

Let us place the pathology model on hold and instead consider being older as an opportunity for continuing growth and development.

Learning to listen

A distinction is made between listening and hearing by suggesting that listening is active and hearing is often passive. Riemen (1986) describes existential presence as follows:

> It is an undeniable fact that there are some people who reveal themselves as 'present'—that is to say, at our disposal—when we are in pain or need to confide in someone, while there are other people who do not give this feeling, however great is their goodwill...The most attentive listener may give me the impression of not being present; he gives me nothing, he cannot make room for me in himself whatever the material favours he is prepared to grant me. The truth is there is a way of listening which is of giving, and another way which is of refusing...Presence is something that reveals itself immediately and unmistakably in a look, a smile, an intonation, or a handshake. (Rieman 1986, p 35)

Riemen suggests that listening to people is an act of participation, and manifests itself as an 'existential presence', whereas hearing implies that words are heard, but not necessarily with full appreciation of what matters or what is important to people in our care.

Seventy per cent of people admitted to the acute care sector are older people. In response to a question about what it is like to be in hospital, Ada, an older patient, replied:

It was my first time in hospital and six women died while I was there. I found that difficult emotionally. One woman died just after I had been talking with her. I cried. One of the young nurses said to me, 'What are you crying for?' I explained that I was upset because that lady had just died. 'How do you know she has died', she said. I answered that I was aware of these things. The nurse said, 'Well I don't know what you are crying for, you don't even know her'. That made me feel worse. It was the younger ones there, the untrained ones. It was as if they thought, 'You are old and you are going to die anyway'. They didn't treat people very well, not as human beings anyway. I had never seen anyone die before. I was very, very upset. And the nurses appeared so matter of fact. I couldn't understand how they could be so cold. First I thought they were not caring, later I thought you have to be tough to be a nurse. (Koch 1993)

Ada's comment shows us what this older woman thinks of nurses, and how she felt depersonalised by their attitude to her. Ada's account of life in the hospital reveals how nurses often do not understand the way people experience healthcare. We do not ask patients routinely about their experience, and often nurses do not listen to what patients say. Talk and listen to find out more about the person who is in your care.

Who is likely to receive nursing care? It is interesting to know that from 2,370,878 people, 85 per cent of older people are living their lives just like you and me. Only 6 per cent of older people need nursing care and mostly they live in nursing homes, where the majority of residents have dementia. Another 11 per cent may live in the community; they may be frail older people, people whose cognitive skills are impaired through early dementia, people with disabilities and people with chronic health conditions. This group of people face many challenges in living as independently as possible in their own homes and communities. Often their needs are complex, and the health services that can meet them may be hard to find. This group are likely to have difficulty managing without assistance.

Helping older people to navigate the health system may be part of the nurse's role. If you find yourself in a clinical placement in the community, you may accompany a district or community nurse in their provision of care. As stated earlier, the largest group of people receiving home care are older people. Complex needs can be either ongoing or short term, based on health conditions or living situation. Expert nursing skills are required to deal with the complexities, but what is paramount is to listen to what the older person has to say. How else can you support them in the provision of nursing care?

Becoming a nurse at the beginning of the twenty-first century means realising that the majority of patients, clients and the community are likely to be older people. Treating older people as individuals, building relationships, sharing your knowledge and helping people navigate the healthcare system requires exceptional nursing skills.

Resources

Australian Bureau of Statistics (ABS): <www.abs.gov.au>. *Follow the* Themes *link to 'Ageing', and to' Disability, Ageing and Carers'.*
Aged and Community Services Australia (formerly Aged Care Australia): <www.agedcare.org.au>. *Fact sheets on topics of health, Medicare, hospitals, residential care, housing.*
Alzheimer's Association NSW: <www.alznsw.asn.au>. *35 practical help sheets.*
Australian Institute of Health and Welfare: Older Australia at a glance, 3rd edn, 2002. Online. Available <http://www.aihw.gov.au/publications/welfare/oag03/index.html>. *38 topics can be downloaded, providing an overview of the health, wellbeing and social circumstances of older Australians, and their health and aged care/welfare services. Information and statistics is included on demography, families and caring, housing, income, retirement, voluntary activities, older people's organisations and expenditure trends. Sources of the data used are given, and further reading suggested. Another link,<www.aihw.gov.au/agedcare/publications/index.html>, takes you to other AIHW publications on ageing and aged care.*
Carers Association Australia: <http://www.carersaustralia.com.au>. *Resources and fact sheets on a variety of topics useful to carers, and details of those available through state carers' associations—look under 'Information and Resources'.*
Commonwealth Department of Health and Aged Care: <http://www. health.gov.au/acc/>. *(a) Australian health and ageing system—the*

concise factbook, 5th edn, June 2005: *a series of regular publications presenting the key statistical indicators of the Australian health and ageing system. (b) Aged and community care publications (some of which can be downloaded or printed using Adobe Acrobat Reader). (c) The Aged Care Hotline can be contacted on 1800 500 853.*
Multicultural Health Communication Service, NSW: <http://mhcs. health.nsw.gov.au/health-public-affairs/mhcs/publications/Older_ People.html>. *This site takes you to the ageing topics from a database of publications, which can be viewed, downloaded and printed in languages other than English.*

References

Koch T 1993 Toward fourth generation evaluation: listening to the voices of older patients: a hermeneutic inquiry. PhD thesis, Manchester University, UK.
Koch T, Power C & Kralik D 2005 100 years old: 24 centenarians tell their stories. Viking/Penguin, London.
Rieman D 1986 Caring and non-caring in the clinical setting: patients' descriptions. Topics in Clinical Nursing:30–36.

6.14 Palliative care

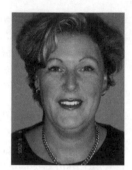

Amanda Johnson

Amanda Johnson
Lecturer, School of Nursing, College of Health and
Science, University of Western Sydney

Your personal experiences of death and the initial experiences of caring for a person dying and their family will shape the future way in which you provide palliative care. The following discussion in this section is designed to support you as you participate in the care of the dying person and her or his family across a range of healthcare settings.

Many nursing students view this type of clinical experience as stressful and challenging as they witness the need to meet the often complex and changing needs of someone who is dying and that person's family. This can seem daunting, frightening, confronting and a somewhat highly anxiety-provoking learning experience, yet the potential for personal and professional growth it offers is exponential.

Current thinking sees a broadening of palliative care principles to embrace not only cancer-oriented illnesses but any life-threatening disease. This means that nurses, as the largest group of health professionals, will need to provide palliative care as a core part of their practice across a range of healthcare settings. Nursing in this context sees the nurse engage holistically with a dying person and his or her family. This active involvement will promote deeper and more meaningful learning.

Learning opportunities

The learning gained during placement will allow you to view death as a normal part of the life cycle and will help you to understand the following:

- the profound effect on the individual and family
- the nurse's role as part of an interdisciplinary team
- the contribution made by a range of allied and health professionals in the management of symptoms
- the selection of interventions that will support the individual's quality of life
- participation in the closure that occurs at someone's death
- death as a positive experience.

Preparing for the placement

Undertaking the following strategies will assist you to prepare for this clinical placement. They will enable you to more actively participate and feel confident in the learning experience.

- Read the recommended text given at the end of this section.
- Write down your feelings about death. Come back to these during the course of the clinical placement and afterwards to see if and how your feelings may or may not have changed. Try to understand what has influenced your thinking in relation to this area of practice.
- Employ self-reflection during and after the clinical experience.
- Identify and write down several self-care strategies you use when stressed. Ensure that these resources are readily available to you during this clinical placement. Remember it is important to care for yourself so that you can provide optimal care.
- Be open to sharing your feelings with other staff (registered nurse, clinical facilitator, nurse educator, nursing unit manager), as this act of sharing validates your own anxieties.

- Find out who else is undertaking a similar clinical placement and establish an informal support network with these peers, as this group often becomes your first contact for support.
- Organise a meeting with your clinical educator before the clinical placement so that you can establish an initial relationship in a neutral zone. This strategy provides an opportunity for you to convey your feelings and anxieties in a less stressful environment and begins to build a trusting relationship with your clinical educator (or other support person, depending on the clinical placement), who will most likely act as a primary support for you.
- Acknowledge that each experience with a dying patient and her or his family will be unique and individual. However, also recognise that there are commonalities, and you will develop competence and confidence in the management of your patients and their families over time.
- Start recording your experiences in a journal. Recounting your stories of caring for dying patients and their families allows you to reflect on and promote learning for future experiences.
- Be open to the expert positive role models present in the clinical placement, as these people will shape your future clinical practice.

Challenges for the student

Understand that the anxiety provoked in this clinical placement is common to many nursing students and is a natural reaction. Acknowledging the types of challenges you may face will help you to manage this anxiety.

These challenges may include the following:

- coping with the physical symptoms and suffering experienced by dying patients

- finding it difficult to talk with those who are dying and their families (knowing how to respond to questions; choosing the 'right' words; knowing how to progress conversations about death; understanding the impact of silence)
- difficulty with the notion of 'being' with people who are dying and their families
- understanding the impact that closure of a relationship with someone who is dying and his or her family has on the nurse
- being scared of not doing the 'right' thing
- understanding the types of deaths and their impact on the nurse
- concerns with physical touch in the care of a dying person
- concerns with the physical preparation of a deceased person

Further reading

Johnson A, Harrison K, Currow D et al 2006 Palliative care and health breakdown. In Chang E, Daly J & Elliott D (eds), Pathophysiology applied to nursing practice, pp 448–471. Elsevier, Sydney.

6.15 Perioperative nursing

Menna Davies
Clinical Nurse Consultant, Operating Suite,
Prince of Wales/Sydney Children's Hospital

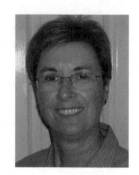

Menna Davies

Perioperative nursing is a challenging, dynamic and exciting specialty area of nursing. The term 'perioperative' relates to the nursing care of the surgical patient immediately before, during and immediately after an operation and offers nurses the opportunity to be involved in a multidisciplinary team caring for a patient during one of the most vulnerable periods of their surgical experience. Within the team, nurses play a vital role in combining technical expertise with fundamental nursing skills and knowledge to ensure patient safety during each phase of the patient's perioperative experience.

In the immediate preoperative phase, nurses assist the anaesthetist in caring for the patient during induction, maintenance and emergence from anaesthesia. The anaesthetic nurse not only provides technical assistance, but emotional care for the patient and, among other attributes, requires good assessment and communication skills.

During the intraoperative phase, the circulating nurse uses aseptic technique to deliver sterile equipment to the operative field. This nurse is also directly involved in maintaining patient safety (for example, by assisting to position the patient and by counting instruments and other items used intraoperatively). The circulating nurse works closely with the instrument nurse, whose role involves preparing the sterile instruments and equipment used by the surgical team. The instrument nurse works closely with the surgeon to provide efficient delivery of instruments and equipment required during the surgical procedure.

Following surgery, the care of the patient is handed over to specialist nurses in the post-anaesthesia recovery unit. These nurses are responsible for closely monitoring the patient's vital signs, as well as managing any complications that may arise during the immediate postoperative period. They provide pain relief and reassurance to the patient and, when the patient is ready to return to the ward area, a detailed handover to the ward staff on the patient's condition.

As this description of the nursing roles indicates, perioperative nurses require a great deal of specialty knowledge to carry out their roles. Depending on the size, complexity of surgery and staffing of an operating suite, nurses may choose to specialise in one of the above roles or may be multiskilled and undertake all the roles described.

Learning opportunities

A clinical placement in a perioperative setting offers the opportunity not only to learn specialty skills and to acquire knowledge and technical expertise, but also to develop skills and knowledge that are transferable to other areas of nursing. For example, it is the most comprehensive anatomy and physiology lesson you will ever receive. Communication, aseptic technique, infection control, patient assessment, pharmacology, pressure area management, airway management, pain management, intravenous fluids and time management are but a few of the topics about which you will learn during a visit to this area. You will also witness a variety of surgical procedures within the ever-changing world of surgery where no two days are ever the same.

Collaboration between educational institutions and health facilities provides undergraduate/trainee enrolled nurses with opportunities for undertaking clinical placements in the perioperative environment. The placements vary from a few days to several weeks, with some educational institutions offering structured elective placements in their programs. Even if a clinical placement is not available, it may be possible to arrange day visits during placements on a surgical ward or to follow a surgical patient through their perioperative experience.

Following registration/enrolment, many hospitals provide structured programs for newly qualified RNs and ENs. Many of these programs include the opportunities for placements in the perioperative environment lasting 3–12 months. During the placement a comprehensive orientation is provided, together with structured learning programs in many facilities. If you decide on a career in perioperative nursing, there are postgraduate/enrolment courses that provide you with the specialist knowledge to further enhance your clinical practice in this specialty area.

If you decide, following a clinical placement, that a career in perioperative nursing is not for you, the understanding you have gained of the patient's perioperative experience will greatly assist you in caring for the surgical patient in the ward and elsewhere. Career opportunities for perioperative nurses can extend beyond the operating theatre into radiology departments, where greater interventional procedures are being carried out, day-only surgery departments, and military and humanitarian organisations.

Perioperative nurses in Australia are very active in state/territory professional organisations and are represented nationally by the Australian College of Operating Room Nurses (ACORN). The college is active in developing standards of care for perioperative settings and provides perioperative nurses with a voice at state and national levels of government. Visit <www.acorn.org.au> to learn more about perioperative nursing opportunities in your state/territory.

6.16 Private hospital nursing

Deánne Grolimund
Learning and Development Manager,
Sydney Adventist Hospital

Margaret Mason
Clinical Nurse Educator,
Sydney Adventist Hospital

Lynette Saul
Clinical Nurse Educator,
Sydney Adventist Hospital

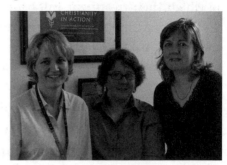

From left to right, Deánne Grolimund,
Margaret Mason and Lynette Saul

Private hospitals are influential on the broader Australian health system. One of their major contributions is in the area of education and training of nurses. The majority of private hospitals in Australia have some form of affiliation with a university. The Australian Private Hospitals Association (2005) reports that an estimated 4000 nurses employed in private hospitals were actively involved in providing nursing education and training in private hospitals in 2004. Private hospitals have continued to support this commitment to training and education because of the associated positive outcomes. It is generally agreed that training and education improves the quality of healthcare. Other benefits include improvement of the work environment, recruitment and retention of staff (Australian Private Hospitals Association 2005).

Private hospitals in Australia have a strong commitment to the implementation and contribution of 'best practice' nursing standards. These facilities promote a culture that embraces professional development and a dedication to quality customer service. All patients wish to be informed and consulted about the nature of their treatment. In a private hospital the patients are empowered by having chosen not only the medical specialist but also the facility in which their treatment will be delivered. The private sector takes pride in providing the latest technology and an aesthetically pleasing environment.

Private hospitals are a viable alternative for students seeking clinical experiences. Learning opportunities similar to those offered in the public sector are available in most private hospitals.

Getting the most out of clinical placement at a private hospital

Be prepared

Preparation for your placement is the key not only to greater understanding but also to increased confidence in your clinical experience:

- Know what your educational institution's course objectives are for your placement.
- Formulate your personal goals.
- Know what you need to do and see. If you are clear about what is required, you can use your learning opportunities to maximum effect.
- Confirm shift times and rosters. Organise transport and plan to arrive early or on time.
- Ensure you have appropriate uniform, including footwear and identification.

Kate, a second-year nursing student was very excited about her clinical placement. She wanted to make a good first impression, so she contacted the NUM of her assigned ward and made arrangements to meet her and orient herself to the ward before commencement. This meant she was more at ease and familiar with the environment on her first day.

Be interested and maximise your learning opportunities

Show an interest in what is happening around you. Ask questions. Observe what the registered nurse does. Find out what is happening and why. Research and find out more. You have many resources available to you, starting with experienced registered nurses and midwives. Clinical nurse educators are available in many areas. Many hospitals have comprehensive libraries for your use, as well as access to research learning requirements.

Amy, a third-year student, sought an opportunity to learn more about a procedure by arranging to observe the surgery being performed on her allocated patient. She initiated this learning experience herself, thus enhancing her understanding of her patient's condition and treatment.

Communication

Talk to the nurses in your team. Voicing your needs will enable us to assist you in reaching your expected goals. Expressing your knowledge of a situation will guide the nursing team in understanding your previous experiences and learning needs. Relating to the interdisciplinary team (doctors, physiotherapists, dieticians etc) can be quite daunting. Your clinical placement is a good opportunity to observe and learn how other nurses communicate in various situations.

Effective communication is an essential nursing skill that you develop with experience. Use your clinical experience to improve how you communicate. Focus on developing professional relationships with the patients and their families. This will increase your confidence in caring for them. You will be more able to assess changes in their condition, and also offer comfort and understanding.

Smile often. If you smile at someone, they may smile back. Endorphins are released when you smile, even with a forced smile. These are our natural analgesics. Imagine how this will help your patients to feel better. The whole team will also be influenced if you smile at them.

Use your initiative

Within your set boundaries and limitations of practice you have plenty of scope to use your initiative. It is important to recognise the difference between a patient's needs and wants, as this is imperative in deciding the priority of care. This is a vital component of critical thinking and decision-making. As a team member you will need to help your nursing team so that they then have the opportunity to show you a specialised skill. For example, 'I will help you make the beds, if you can show me that vacuum dressing'.

If you identify a patient need, follow through with action. If the action required is outside your scope of practice, a referral will be required. You can refer to your preceptor, facilitator, the team leader or unit manager. The rewards of teamwork are so much more than sharing the physical loads. You will gain other benefits, as well as the gratitude of your co-workers—your self-worth and job satisfaction will soar.

Be a 'good looker'

Look at your patients and be aware of the whole environment. It is imperative you report and document any and all changes in condition.

Follow policies and procedures

All hospital policies and procedures should be readily available for your use in every clinical area. You are expected to adhere to these at all times. If you are unsure, ask a staff member or your facilitator.

Ben was on clinical placement in a plastics unit caring for a patient. As the patient's doctor left the room, he asked Ben to remove the drain tube. Ben looked up the procedure in the policy and procedure manual and was able to gather the necessary equipment. Ben's initiative ensured he was confident to perform the procedure under the supervision of his grateful and impressed preceptor.

Last but not least—have fun! Spending time in the hospital environment can and should be a positive experience for all.

Reference

Australian Private Hospitals Association (2005) Annual report 2004–2005. Online. Available <http://www.apha.org.au/publications.html>.

6.17 Rural health nursing

Andrew Christopherson
Senior Flight Nurse,
Royal Flying Doctor Service (RFDS)

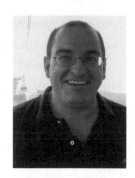

Andrew Christopherson

Congratulations! I hope you are reading this as part of your preparation before a clinical placement in remote, rural or aviation nursing. The better prepared you are for your placement, the more you will gain from it. This overview provides both general and specific advice for students on clinical placement in remote, rural and aviation nursing settings.

Successful placements are based as much on yourself as on the clinical facility. The factors you can best control are attitude, behaviour and appearance. You may have some input into the facility factors, but your control of these is extremely limited as a student.

The attitude you display on and about placement broadcasts your attitude to nursing. Enthusiastic, interested students generally have pleasant clinical placements. If you do have personal or study problems, please seek support sooner rather than later. Students displaying motivational difficulties on clinical placement generally do not do well. A stressful clinical placement may have long-term consequences for your nursing career.

Two areas where your commitment is on display are appearance and behaviour. Most clinical environments have uniform or casual clothing standards. Your personal appearance should meet the facility or organisation standard.

Similarly, your behaviour should display your developing, or even better, your already developed sense of professionalism.

Clinical placements provide opportunities to participate in the professional and social contexts of nursing as well as to give supervised patient care. If you are considering remote, rural or aviation nursing as a career path, placement in these settings as a student is a distinct advantage.

Preparing for the placement

Ideally you should have some theoretical preparation for the clinical setting before placement. If this has not happened, try to obtain some background information about the practice area and to get some idea of current clinical themes and issues.

In any practice area you must also have a clear idea of your scope of supervised practice and your objectives for the placement.

Minimal preparation should cover the following:

- confirmation of the dates for your placement
- the location of your placement
- assessment and evaluation method(s) used
- the start time on the first day
- uniform requirements, if any

If you are travelling to a clinical placement, it is also vital to confirm your travel and accommodation arrangements. Please do not assume that these can always be provided by the clinical facility or organisation.

Remote and rural clinical placements

Clinical practice settings outside metropolitan areas require the flexibility and sense of humour characteristic of remote and rural nursing. The major challenge for students on these placements is often travelling to and from the clinical setting. Once on placement, my experience has been that most students have a rewarding time in remote and rural settings and gain exposure to comprehensive nursing across a diverse range of cultural and client groups.

The best specific hint for these placements is to contact the remote and rural organisation or facility beforehand. Some of the advice and orientation material used for its own staff may also be suitable for your use as background information. This may also include information about transcultural nursing practice and the requirement to deliver nursing care with cultural safety.

Aviation nursing placements

The most important advice for aviation nursing clinical placement is 'safety first'. Safety is paramount in the aviation environment and compliance with safety procedures is enforced with the full power of federal law. Consequently, it is vital that you understand and comply with any safety information provided by the facility or organisation.

Other hints for clinical placement in aviation nursing include the following:

* Space is often limited on board medical aircraft. On some flights you may not be able to accompany the crew because of space and/or weight. If you are 'bumped', please accept this graciously.
* Luggage space is also limited. In civilian aviation nursing aircraft, this limit is often one small bag.
* Some of the aviation nursing practice skills are at an expert or advanced level. Examples of this may include pre-hospital care, triage, midwifery and care of the ventilated patient. Because of scope-of-practice issues, you may not be able to perform these skills yourself, even if supervised.
* Some aspects of aviation nursing may be time-critical. In these cases, mission priorities may take precedence over student education.
* The physical environment can result in a type of fatigue similar to jet lag. Remember to remain hydrated and to present for duty well rested.

Conclusion

Some tips for a successful placement are:

- Aim for competent compassionate patient care.
- Remember that you are a guest at the clinical facility or organisation.
- Aim for professional standards of behaviour, particularly regarding reliability and punctuality.
- Project enthusiasm and commitment.
- Be open to suggestions.
- Apply critical thinking, but voice any criticism very carefully.
- Apply reflective practice to the clinical placement.

6.18 Surgical nursing

Dee Maguire
Surgical Nurse Educator, Westmead Hospital,
Sydney West Area Health Service

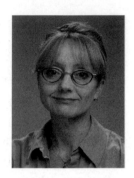

Dee Maguire

Surgical nursing is both a fascinating and diverse domain of clinical practice, involving skills that can easily be transferred to most other specialties. For this reason, surgical nursing is an excellent foundation for your journey into nursing as a career.

The practice setting is primarily one that requires astute assessment and management of the patient both before and after operation. It is the individual patient's response to surgery, anaesthesia and intervention that dictates the recovery period. Therefore, skilful and diligent assessment is paramount in the detection of potential postoperative complications that may have an impact on the ideal recovery for each patient. Modern techniques in minimally invasive surgery have reduced the length of stay (LOS) and facilitated earlier discharge. Monitoring the patient through the surgical experience also involves early patient education and individual discharge planning from the outset. For this reason, the surgical nurse is not just a specialist but also a generalist who is flexible, creative and broadly skilled.

Learning opportunities

Within this context of diversity, the student nurse will be exposed to a rich and stimulating learning terrain. You will explore not only the advances in surgical techniques and the affect of these on the patient, but also what anatomical structures were involved during surgery. For this reason, you will constantly refer to your knowledge of anatomy and physiology, which builds the platform for your clinical practice. You will see several venous access devices and it will be important for you to know the purpose of these lines and their distinguishing features. You will see complex wounds and learn which type of dressing is appropriate and at what stage during the healing process it is required (for example, vacuum-assisted wound closure). You will see a range of wound drainage systems that promote wound healing, and you will be taught the principles of monitoring and safe drain removal. The surgical pace, most importantly, will prepare you to think on your feet and to critically problem-solve quickly and effectively.

You will be encouraged to link patient diagnosis with the type of specialty surgery performed, and then relate this to the specifics of the patient. Only by obtaining the 'whole picture' will you be informed about individual response to surgery. An excellent method of doing this is to follow a patient from the preoperative stage through to discharge (this would include being an observer during surgery). You might like to start with a field of surgery that interests you, such as vascular, plastics or hepatobiliary, then reinforce your knowledge by reading current research on that specialty. By following the patient through her or his personal experience you will be in a strong position to make these links between the person and the surgery. Your specific knowledge will extend beyond the surgery to 'how' the patient responded. Questions you could ask yourself during the case study include: did the patient have any intraoperative complications; how was the patient's pain managed; did any regular medication need reviewing post-surgery? These are just a few examples; you can think of many more.

Preparing for the placement

Before venturing into this exciting domain, some of your preparation will include gathering a schema about the general principles in pre- and postoperative care. These will include preoperative assessment and legal consent, the importance of referring to specific postoperative orders, pain management, fluid status and resuscitation, prevention of post-surgery complications (for example, deep vein thrombosis, wound infection and atelectasis).

After establishing a general picture, move on to reviewing a couple of surgical procedures for each specialty; for example, for vascular surgery you might look at abdominal aortic aneurysm (AAA) and femoral popliteal bypass. This is useful because, despite differences in surgery, there are generic principles that cross all specialties. You will also need to know the difference between septic and hypovolaemic shock, and their key indicators.

It is also very important to consistently make references to each body system while learning about surgery. If a patient has a thyroidectomy, for example, you will need to understand exactly what the thyroid does and what will happen when that gland is removed. In effect, your knowledge of body systems will be a giant pool, which you will constantly dip into during your placement in surgery. Your knowledge will actually become activated!

Best wishes and good luck with your career.

Recommended reading

Manley K & Bellman L 2000 Surgical nursing: advancing practice. Churchill Livingstone, London.
Pudner R 2005 Nursing the surgical patient, Chapters 9, 11–18, 20–22. Baillère-Tindall, Edinburgh.

Glossary

Accountability
Relates to the forms of responsibility and duty, and to the notion of 'being in charge of' in nursing practice.

Acculturation
The individual's adaptation to the customs, values, beliefs and behaviours of a new culture.

Acuity
The degree of complexity of a patient's state of illness and the level of care required.

Advocacy
A critical function of the nursing role that incorporates the ethical principle of beneficence, defending the rights of others or acting on their behalf.

Ageism
Prejudice against the older adult that perpetuates negative stereotyping of ageing as a period of decline.

Androgogy
The art and science of helping adults learn; a term coined by Malcolm Knowles to describe his theory of adult learning.

Assess
To gather, summarise and interpret relevant data about a learner or patient to make a decision or plan.

Australian Nursing and Midwifery Council (ANMC)
A national organisation established for the purpose of facilitating a national approach to the regulation of nursing and midwifery in Australia. The ANMC works with state and territory nurse and midwife regulatory authorities to develop standards for regulation and to provide a collective voice for these authorities.

Australian Nursing and Midwifery Council Competency Standards for the Registered Nurse (2005)
A national benchmark for registered nurses that reinforces responsibility and accountability in delivering quality nursing care through safe and effective work practice. The competencies are organised into four domains: Professional Practice, Critical Thinking and Analysis, Provision and Coordination of Care, and Collaborative and Therapeutic Practice.

Best practice
The use of high-quality clinical evidence to inform and underpin patient care decisions and nursing actions.

Clinical educator
The registered nurse assigned to facilitate the learning of students. A clinical educator is usually allocated to a group of students, and may or may not be employed by the educational institution. Also called facilitator, clinical teacher and nurse teacher.

Clinical governance
A system of management that encourages openness about strengths and weaknesses, and that incorporates the need to be proactive through best practice to promote excellence in healthcare.

Clinical learning environment
The placement location in a healthcare facility where nursing students are allocated in order to achieve objectives, care for clients/patients and undertake assigned learning activities.

Clinicians
The nurses working with patients/clients in the clinical learning environment.

Code of Ethics for Nurses in Australia
A framework that outlines the nursing profession's intention to accept the rights of individuals and to uphold these rights in practice. The code provides guidelines for ethical practice and identifies the fundamental moral commitments of the nursing profession.

Code of Professional Conduct for Nurses in Australia
A set of national standards of nursing conduct for nurses in Australia that identifies the minimum requirements for conduct in the profession.

Competence
The combination of knowledge, skills, behaviours, attitudes, values and abilities that underpin effective and/or superior performance in a professional/occupational area.

Compliance
Submission or yielding to regimens or practices prescribed or established by others.

Confidentiality
A binding social contract or covenant; a professional obligation to respect privileged information between health provider and client.

Cultural competence
The ability to demonstrate knowledge and understanding of another person's culture, and accept and respect cultural differences by adapting interventions to be congruent with that specific culture when delivering care.

Culture
A complex concept that is an integral part of each person's life. It includes knowledge, beliefs, values, morals, customs, traditions and habits acquired by the members of a society.

Disability
Inability to perform some key functions of living.

Duty
Responsibility; professional expectation.

Educational institution
An institution that provides an accredited nursing program. The institution may be a university, school of nursing, or college.

Educator
The teaching role a nurse assumes in supporting, encouraging and assisting the learner.

Enrolled nurse
A person licensed to provide nursing care under the supervision of a registered nurse. Each state or territory in Australia licenses nurses separately.

Ethical dilemma
A problem in which there is a moral or ethical choice to be made between choices that seem equally unfavourable.

Ethics
Guiding principles of human behaviour; morals.

Ethnicity
A dynamic and complex concept referring to how members of a group perceive themselves and how, in turn, they are perceived by others in relation to the population subgroup's common heritage of customs, characteristics, language and history.

Ethnocentrism
Belief that one's own culture is superior and all other cultures are less sophisticated.

Feedback
Valid and reliable judgments about students' performance for the purposes of recognising strengths and areas for improvement. Feedback provides students with information about what they are expected to do and how they are progressing. Ideally it is provided about all activities or situations in which the student has been involved.

Healthcare facility
An institution where the delivery of healthcare is the primary focus. Examples include hospitals, outpatient clinics, medical centres and extended care facilities. These may be publicly or privately operated.

Healthcare team
An interdisciplinary group of healthcare professionals and non-professionals who provide services to patients and their families in an attempt to maximise the optimal health and wellbeing of the person to whom their activities are directed.

Horizontal violence
Covert or overt dissatisfaction directed by nurses towards one another and towards those less powerful than themselves. Usually it is the nurses in the least organisationally powerful positions that manifest bullying among themselves and towards those with even less power.

Interdisciplinary healthcare team
The different disciplinary groups of people responsible for working as a team to provide high-quality healthcare to patients.

International nursing student
A student undertaking an approved nursing course or program who is not an Australian citizen and is not permanently residing in Australia.

Learning objectives
Intended outcomes of the educational process that are action-oriented rather than content-oriented, and learner-centred rather than teacher-centred.

Mentor
A nurse who supports a nursing student during placement experience. The nurse takes responsibility for supervising, directly or indirectly, the student's practice. Sometimes referred to as a preceptor, buddy/professional partner/allocated registered nurse.

Negligence
Doing or not doing an act, pursuant to a duty, that a reasonable person in the same circumstances would or would not do, and that results in injury to another person.

Patient-centred care
A way of practising that focuses on an individual's personal beliefs, values, wants, needs and desires. An approach in which patients' freedom to make their own decisions is recognised as a fundamental and valuable human right.

Privacy
A right for all individuals that protects their personal information and the dissemination of such information.

Reflection
A process by which nurses process their clinical experience and their understanding of what they are doing and why they are doing it, and consider the impact it has on themselves and others. Reflection promotes learning from practice through exploration, questioning and growing through, and as a consequence of, clinical experiences.

Registered nurse
A person who is licensed to practice nursing in Australia (as approved by each state or territory Act).

Scope of practice
A framework of nursing activities that particular nurses are educated, competent and authorised to perform within a specific context.

Sexual harassment
Conduct of a sexual nature that is unwanted and unwelcome by the receiver. Conduct is considered unwelcome when it is neither invited nor solicited and the behaviour is deemed offensive and undesirable.

Student
A student of nursing may be an undergraduate nursing student or a trainee enrolled nurse.

Undergraduate nursing program
An initial program of study that leads to the award of a Bachelor degree. Provided at institutions of higher education (usually universities, but may be institutes or approved colleges).

Index